colour**me**beautiful

colour me
CONFIDENT

change your look – change your life!

Veronique Henderson and Pat Henshaw

hamlyn

This book is dedicated
to Miriam Hyman

An Hachette Livre UK Company

First published in Great Britain in 2006 by
Hamlyn, a division of Octopus Publishing Group Ltd
2–4 Heron Quays, London E14 4JP

www.octopusbooks.co.uk

Text Copyright © 2006 colour me beautiful

Design Copyright © 2006 Octopus Publishing Group Ltd

Every effort has been made to reproduce the colours
in this book accurately, however the printing process
can lead to some discrepancies. The colour samples
provided should be used as a guideline only.

ISBN: 978-0-600-61395-4

A CIP catalogue record for this book
is available from the British Library

Printed and bound in China

10 9 8 7 6 5 4

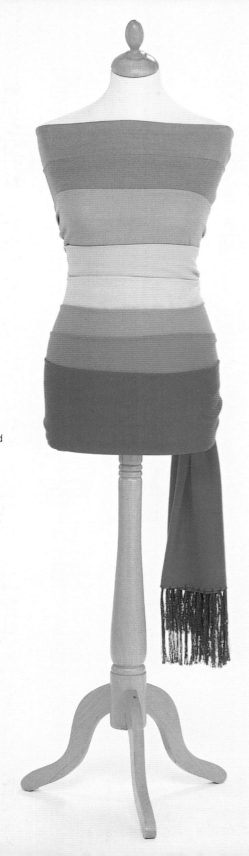

colour me
CONFIDENT

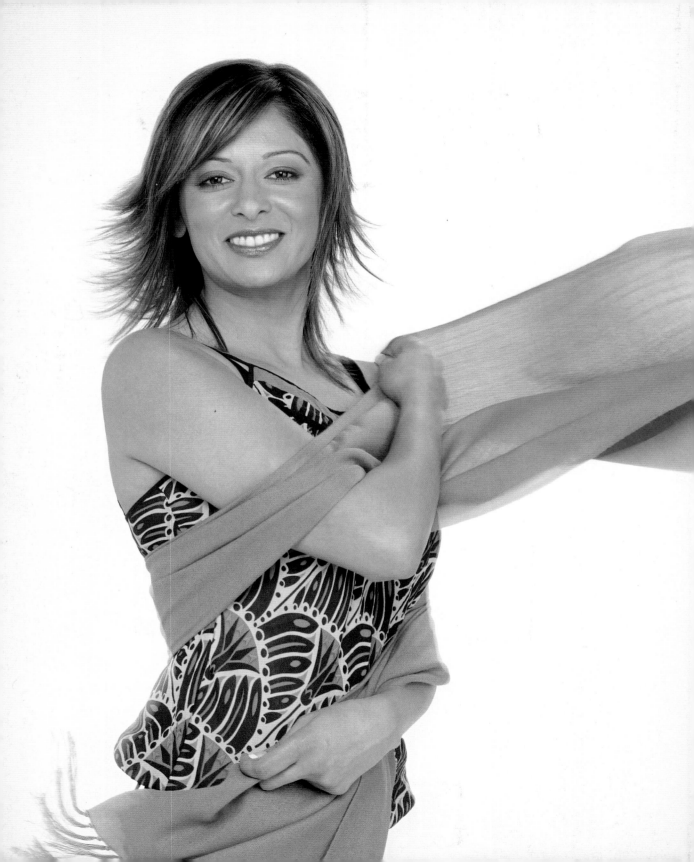

Contents

Introduction

Of the many ways in which we choose to express ourselves, the colour and style of our clothes probably make the most immediate and powerful impact. Clothes do not simply cover the body and protect us from the elements – they make a visual statement about how we view ourselves. Clothes reinforce our self-image and help to define who we are. They can boost our confidence when we know we look good, but when we get it wrong they can sap that confidence just as quickly.

'The badly dressed woman, people remember the clothes. With a well-dressed woman, they remember the woman.' Coco Chanel

Managing your appearance is an important part of who you are. It tells people about your personality and your lifestyle. Nobody can deny that, in today's world, image matters. We are bombarded with perfect images of actresses and models, and more and more emphasis is placed upon looking the part and dressing for success. We all make quick assessments based on how people look. And, while making a judgement on limited information is not the best way to go, it is important to acknowledge that clothing and personal appearance are a form of communication.

Being well dressed does not have to mean dressing expensively or being at the cutting edge of fashion. According to **colour me beautiful**, there are five key points that define a well-dressed woman. Your clothes should:

Complement your colouring
Flatter your body lines, scale and proportions
Be appropriate
Match your style personality
Look current

Whatever your budget, the fashion choices are endless. While increased choice can be exciting, it can also be overwhelming and confusing. When it comes to choosing your wardrobe, the key is to know and understand why some pieces work better than others. Forget those fashion faux-pas languishing in your wardrobe and look forward to understanding what is special about you.

Clothes are wonderful tools that you can manipulate to present yourself to advantage, regardless of your size and proportions. By recognizing your physical assets – and limitations – you can explore the many ways in which clothing can be used to draw attention, to conceal, to camouflage and to create optical illusions. In addition, we are all individuals with a personal style that governs the way we wear our hair, apply make-up and tie a scarf around our neck.

All about **colour me beautiful**

For more than 25 years, **colour me beautiful** has been the world's leading image consultancy. Millions of women, including the ubiquitous Bridget Jones, have benefited from 'having their colours done'. Since the company started in Virginia, USA, in 1978, and the European arm in London in 1983, a small army of image consultants have had the opportunity to learn first-hand just what works for women and how women perceive their image. Based on this unique insight, the company has developed and refined its advice from the original and simple 'four seasons' approach to colour to a more sophisticated approach that encompasses every aspect of your personal image. While colour will always be a central theme, it is only part of the story in terms of developing a personal image and style. You can enjoy taking a fresh look at how to wear colours, rather than simply learning what colours you should wear.

The consultants at **colour me beautiful**, some of whom are featured in this book, come from all walks of life. Many had other careers before they trained with the organization. They bring with them their collective experiences that make **colour me beautiful** the world's largest and most successful image consultancy. Other women featured in this book have experienced the **colour me beautiful** concept for the first time. They all have one thing in common – they are now confident women.

In addition to working with real women all over the world, **colour me beautiful** has developed programmes for clothes stores, as personal shopping has become a popular service for many small and large retailers. A specialist team of consultants also work within commerce and industry on the importance of image in business; they even help members of the motor trade to sell cars to women. In recent years many consumer goods companies have seen the benefit of adding the services of **colour me beautiful** to their promotional campaigns, particularly when colour is involved.

Not a day goes by without a call to the London headquarters from the national press, TV or radio requesting information on colour, image and fashion. The questions are varied: Will this new colour work for a world class football team? What do you make of this film star's shoes? So, when it comes to colour, style, make-up and staying current, you are undoubtedly in good hands.

Why buy this book?

The aim of this book is to help you to identify the best colours for you to wear and to acknowledge your body lines, scale and proportion. Armed with this knowledge, together with a sense of your 'style personality', you will have the confidence to build a wardrobe that is practical, professional and/or as glamorous as you need it to be. You will learn that, to meet the demands of your lifestyle, your wardrobe does not have to bulge; it just needs balance. It will become easy for you to shop efficiently, to avoid disaster purchases and to enjoy yourself more in the process.

Basically, you want a wardrobe that works for you. There are many demands on our lives and having clothes suitable for all occasions can often be beyond our budget and against our inclinations. A co-ordinated wardrobe takes a little planning, forethought and a strong will to avoid impulse buys. Following the guidelines given in this book will keep you on the straight and narrow without taking the fun out of shopping (for those of you who enjoy it) and without making it a torment (for those who don't).

The right selection of clothes will not only make you look great physically but also help you to feel good about yourself – and therefore you become more confident. Wearing the right colours and flattering styles can put a smile on your face, lift your spirits and improve your outlook.

How does this book work?

This book is not about changing your physical appearance (though sometimes a little exercise and diet might help). It will not recommend liposuction, botox or any sort of surgery. The aim is to bring out the best in you, just as the team of **colour me beautiful** consultants around the world have done every day over the past 25 years for millions of happy, confident women from all walks of life.

Does your lifestyle allow you the time and budget to visit the hairdresser twice a week? Can you spend a fortune on clothes? Do you have endless time to go shopping for clothes while juggling a full-time job, children, a partner, a dog, a garden and a social life? In this book you will get hints and tips on how to make the most of yourself with the minimal effort and budget.

The heart of the book guides you to your dominant colour palette – be it light, deep, warm, cool, clear or soft – then fine-tunes it to the secondary characteristic – warm or cool, soft or clear. Armed with your palette of colours, you are encouraged to assess and learn more about your shape, your proportions and your 'style personality' and to choose and wear your clothes accordingly, and with confidence.

Why **colour me beautiful**?

It will give you confidence

✓ Wearing the right colour and style of clothes will make you look younger and healthier.

✓ Knowing how to adapt your wardrobe for different lifestyles increases your self-esteem (as well as making the most of your purchases).

✓ By adapting your look, staying current and developing your own individual style, you will feel more confident.

> Once you know you look good, you are ready to face the world – or any situation that calls for poise and control

It will make you unique
No two women will have exactly the same colouring, size and shape, scale and proportion, personality or budget. But It's useful to have some guidelines to help you make sense of all the choices and focus on who you are and what you really need.

Your unique style – the way you wear your hair, your clothes and how they reflect your lifestyle – is dictated by your personality. With the help of **colour me beautiful**, you stay the same you – but become more confident.

It will help you make the most of your shape
All women wish for the perfect body but, unfortunately, nature is not always as kind as we would like. With some simple tricks and tips from **colour me beautiful**, any woman can improve her appearance regardless of her size.

It will help you to shop successfully
With so many demands on our lives, having suitable clothes for every occasion can often be beyond our reach. With a little forethought and some willpower, you will learn to avoid impulse and unwise buys, and have a wardrobe that works all year round. By following some simple guidelines, the days of a wardrobe full of clothes but nothing to wear will be gone. Learn the secrets that **colour me beautiful** clients discover every day in consultants' studios.

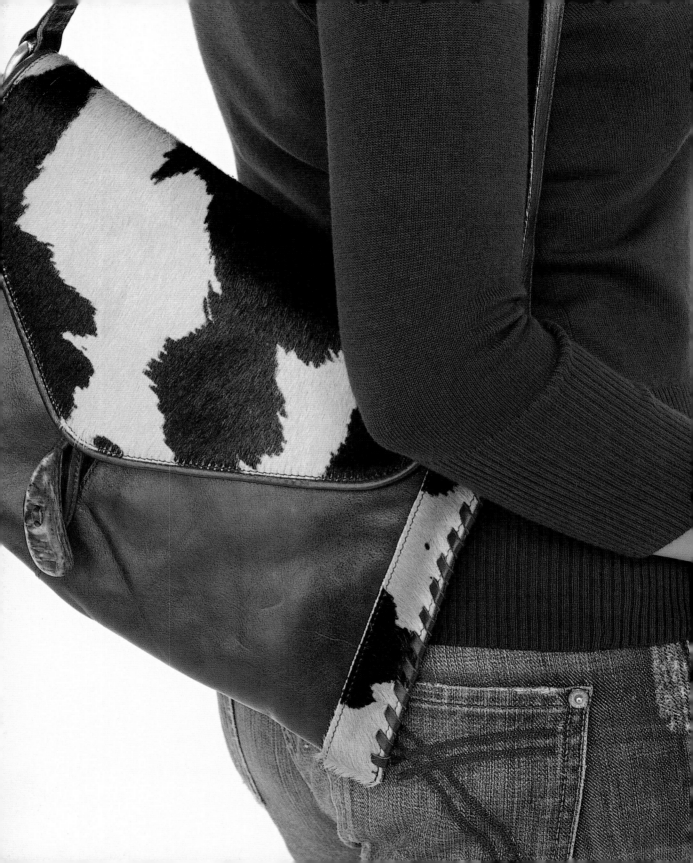

1
time for a change

Take a fresh look

For whatever reason – perhaps a new job, your children leaving home or meeting a new partner – there are periods in every woman's life when the clothes that always seemed right just don't do the job any more. This is the time to take a fresh look at yourself and to develop a style that is uniquely your own.

Every day you meet new people, and some of them may become friends, even enemies. Do you feel confident when you meet someone for the first time? Only 7 per cent of a person's judgement of you is based on what you say to them. The rest of their judgement is based on your appearance and body language. So, when you are getting ready to meet new people, do you know exactly what to wear, or do you end up with a pile of clothes on the bedroom floor and wearing your old favourites? Try this confidence test.

The confidence test

Stand (fully dressed) in front of the mirror, then:
1 **Look at yourself**
2 **Smile**
3 **Pay yourself a compliment**

If you find this easy to do, then congratulations. It is more likely, however, that you will have found only faults: that you're not tall enough/your legs are too short/your hair is lifeless. But how many women who wish for longer legs actually have wonderful long bodies? Likewise, some women may complain that their waists are too big, even though they invariably have small bottoms and hips. This book will help you start to look at yourself in a new, more positive way.

> Did you know that when you meet someone for the first time you have only 30 seconds to make a lasting impression?

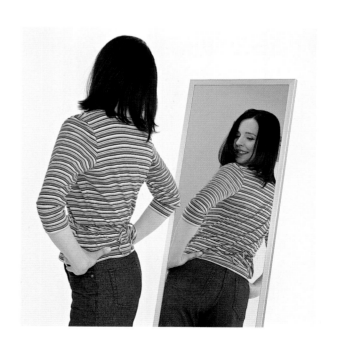

Start by filling in the questionnaire below:

Things I like about myself

....
....
....

Things I'd like to change

....
....
....

About colours

☐ Do you wear the same colours every day?

☐ Are there colours that you wear only at the weekend?

☐ Are you afraid of colour?

☐ Do you tend to wear only black?

About shopping

☐ Do you dislike shopping?

☐ Do you have a wardrobe full of clothes but nothing to wear?

☐ Do you need a different wardrobe for work?

About make-up and grooming

☐ Have you been applying your make-up in the same way for years?

☐ Have you had the same hairstyle for more than three years?

Whatever you have ticked are the issues on which you need to focus. For advice on colour: *go to pages 20–105*; for help with your wardrobe: *go to pages 178–189*; for make-up and grooming tips: *go to pages 156–177*.

How to use this book

You are not going to change your look in an instant. Instead, you will find that you will use this book as a manual that you will dive into over a period of time. Once you have identified your priorities from the questionnaire on the previous page, make one of them your starting point. Take it step by step and be confident with each stage – colour, make-up, style and accessories. Often, **colour me beautiful** clients will attend a colour session and then come back a month later for the style session. Revisiting a concept will give you a fuller understanding and the confidence to go ahead and use your new-found insight.

There is no miracle solution. While there are some easy tips that will give instant answers, you may need time to take other advice on board. In all cases you have to start with your existing wardrobe – a tweak here and there may be all that is needed – and what your budget allows. Your ultimate aim is to become a confident person who knows how to make the most of herself and who will not hesitate to make a choice when facing her wardrobe every morning.

Making a change

Step 1 – decision time

✓ Identify the need for change.

✓ Prepare yourself for a challenge.

Step 2 – colour

✓ Colour makes the initial impact, so find out what colours are perfect for you. See Chapter 2, Choosing the right colours for you: *go to pages 20–105*.

✓ By understanding how colour is made up, you will see how colours look together and work best to flatter you: *go to pages 22–23*.

✓ Read about the science of colour to understand that although you will have 42 recommended colours, these, in fact, represent thousands of colours that you can wear: *go to pages 24–25*.

Step 3 – style

✓ Take a long look at yourself to establish your basic body shape: *go to pages 108–111*.

✓ Scale and proportion matter too – and this book shows you why: *go to pages 130–132*.

✓ From your neck to your ankles, analyse every detail of your body: *go to pages 134–137*.

✓ Identify your style personality and learn how to enhance it: *go to pages 138–155*.

✓ Learn which fabrics and textures flatter your body shape – they can make or break an outfit: *go to pages 112–125*.

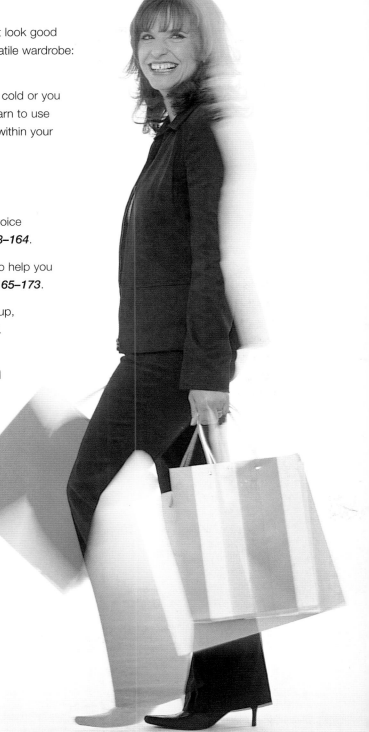

Step 4 – shopping habits

✓ Learn how to shop effectively for clothes that look good on you and go together, thus creating a versatile wardrobe: **go to pages 178–189**.

✓ Whether the thought of shopping leaves you cold or you come to life in the shopping mall, you can learn to use shopping time wisely and to shop efficiently within your budget: **go to pages 182–183**.

Step 5 – your face

✓ Assess your face shape to make the best choice of hairstyle and spectacles: **go to pages 158–164**.

✓ Follow the make-up application techniques to help you put together a groomed look: **go to pages 165–173**.

✓ Take notes from the expert advice on make-up, hair and accessories: **go to pages 156–177**.

Step 6 – putting it into action

✓ Pulling it all together: colour + body shape + scale + proportion + styling personality + accessories + budget = the real you.

With sound advice for real women, backed by years of experience from the top **colour me beautiful** team, this book will show you how to achieve the top-to-toe makeover that will give you confidence and change your life. It's up to you now.

The well-dressed woman

Why is image so important? Because, as we have seen, in every walk of life we are judged by our appearance. When you feel good, you are more confident, you stand straighter, you smile more and you even speak with more conviction.

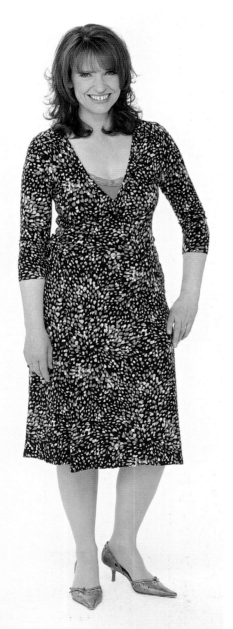

Has anybody ever said to you, 'Are you not feeling well today?' when in fact you are feeling perfectly fit? It may simply be that you are wearing the wrong colour. On the other hand, there may be occasions when you feel tired and stressed but still get complimented. At **colour me beautiful**, we're in the compliment business and we want to make sure that every day you receive compliments about the way YOU look, rather than about the clothes you are wearing.

The key to success

Complement your colouring

Your clothes should work in harmony and balance with the colouring of your skin, hair and eyes. If you are dressed in the right colours, people will see more of you than the clothes you are wearing. Once you understand the right colours and styles for you, you will buy only what suits you when you go shopping. The result will be a more co-ordinated wardrobe.

Flatter your body lines, scale and proportions

You will feel more comfortable wearing clothes that complement your build. An understanding of your basic shape will give you the knowledge to choose clothes that flatter your body line and balance your scale and proportion. For every woman, the aim is to have the appearance of a balanced body.

Choose appropriate clothes

It is important that your clothes reflect your lifestyle, whether it be professional, casual and relaxed or formal – or a combination of all three. Not only should your clothes be appropriate for the occasion, you also need to be comfortable in the style of clothes you wear.

Match your style personality

You will have a preference for a certain style of clothes, the shops you like to buy from and the way you accessorize your look. It is your style personality that will pull together the colours, lines and shape of your clothes.

Look current

Nothing ages a woman more than clothes that are a decade out of fashion. Fads come and go every year but trends stay for at least half a decade. The well-dressed woman understands the trends and may use the fads as fun items in her wardrobe.

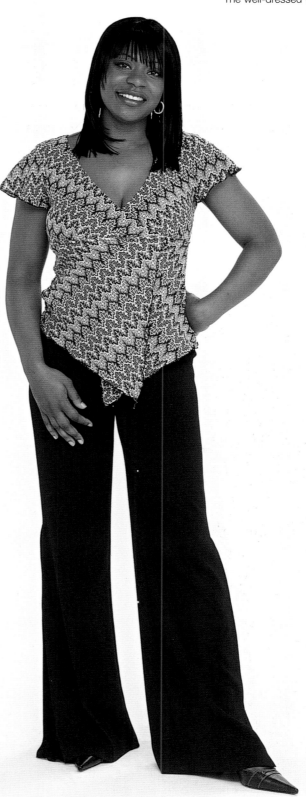

It could be you

Be inspired by these before and after makeovers. Each makeover is the result of a step-by-step process, and through the next few chapters you will see how these women have transformed themselves.

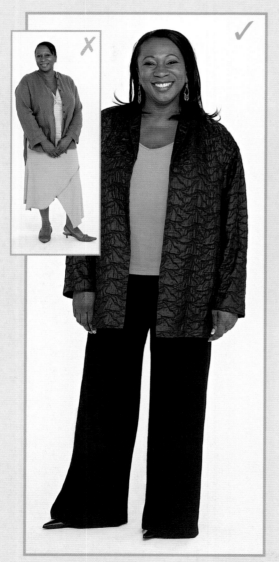

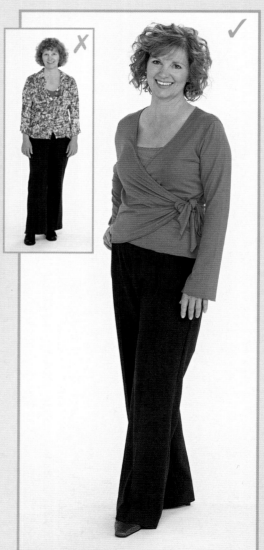

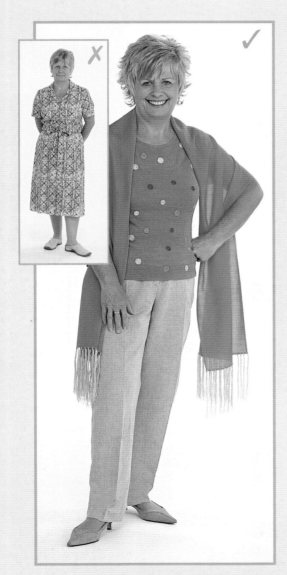

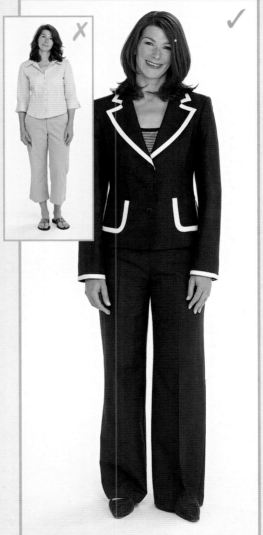

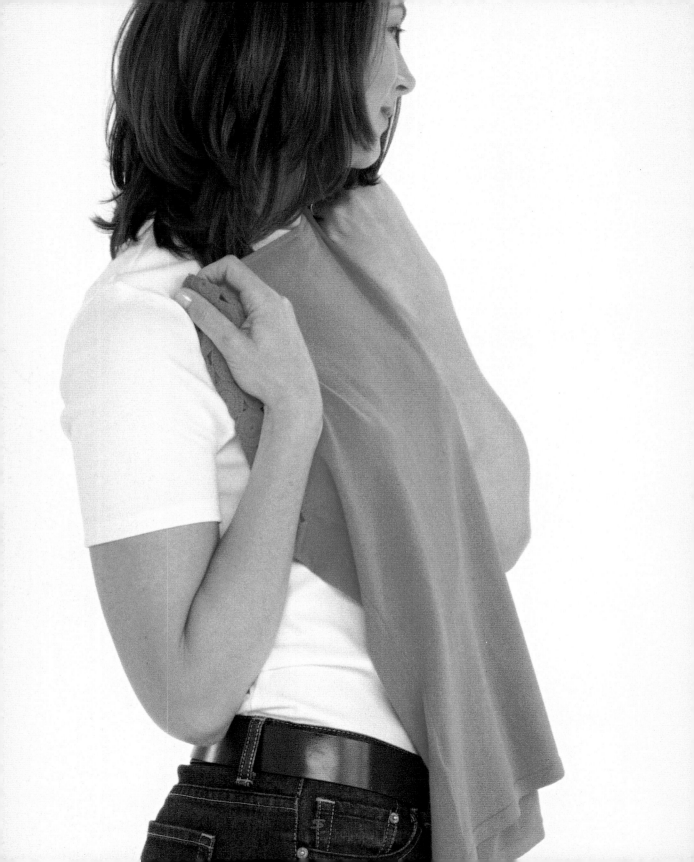

2

choosing the right colours for you

Finding your colours

Colour can be magical. Seeing a flash of colour emerge from a largely monochromatic crowd is energizing, like a breath of fresh air. And once you start wearing colours, there will be no stopping you. For many years neutral colours held sway in fashion but now that colour – in all its hues – is back, the time is right to learn how to make colours work for you. So let us take you on a colourful and stylish journey.

Once you understand your own colouring

✓ Shopping will become easier, the choice of colours second nature.

✓ You will always have in your wardrobe the right combination of colours to wear.

✓ You will gain confidence from knowing that the colours you are wearing are those that flatter.

✓ You will be on the exciting path to a new you.

How colour works

When you wear colour near your face, the light reflects it upwards; this can cast either flattering tones or dark shadows, depending on the mix of the colour and your skin tone. This is one reason why it is important to work out your dominant colouring type and discover which are the right colours for you: *go to pages 34–105*.

There is a psychological aspect to colour, too and the colours you wear can communicate non-verbal messages of various kinds. Soft and light tones, for example, will make you appear approachable and friendly, while a red top in the right shade will help to give you the confidence you need when facing a stressful situation. Colours that you might wear on a first date with a man you wish to impress will probably not be suitable at a school parents' evening, nor at an important business meeting where you want to appear in control: *go to pages 28–31*.

Once you know what your most flattering colours are, it will be time to concentrate on your choice of accessories and make-up: *go to pages 156–177*. No more guesswork and drawers full of scarves and make-up that you do not wear, without knowing exactly why.

Most women wear only
20 per cent of their wardrobe
80 per cent of the time

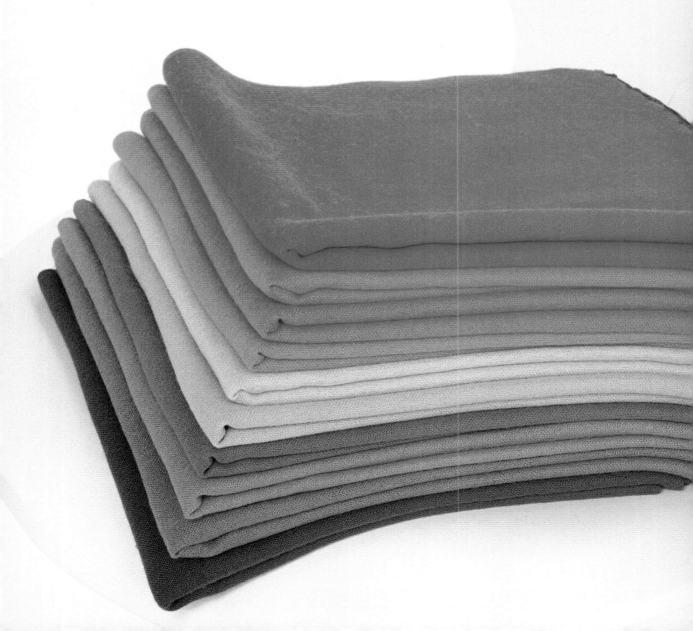

The science of colour

There are two main influences behind **colour me beautiful's** current approach to colour – those of Johannes Itten and Alfred Munsell. The seasonal colour concept that lay behind the original **colour me beautiful** – and which lasted for over 20 years – was first developed in the 1920s by the artist Johannes Itten of the Bauhaus school. Itten noticed that his students always did their best work using colours they had chosen themselves. In his book, *The Art of Colour*, Itten reveals the strong relationship between a student's appearance, their personality and the colours they liked to work with.

This concept was further developed at the Fashion Academy of Los Angeles, founded in 1972. Former student Carole Jackson made the seasonal concept popular in her book, *Color Me Beautiful*, published in 1980. The book was translated into many languages and for months remained on the *New York Times* bestseller list. In 1986 Doris Pooser developed Carole Jackson's seasonal concept further, but with the addition of the Munsell theory (see below), in her book, *Always in Style*.

The Munsell system was partly responsible for **colour me beautiful** moving from four to twelve seasonal palettes in 1991 with the publication of Mary Spillane's *The Complete Style Guide*. Its inclusion in today's **colour me beautiful** approach gives a more flexible way of using colour. The beauty of Munsell's system is that it can be used to describe a person's colouring as well as to specify the colours they should wear, the aim always being to create harmony and balance between the two. The theory behind his system is that all colours have one dominant characteristic and one or two secondary characteristics. A person's colouring will also have one dominant characteristic and, for the purpose of this book, one secondary characteristic. Working with this formula will give women a reliable, versatile and easy-to-follow way of using colour.

The Munsell system

Munsell's is the most widely accepted system of colour measurement; it is used by both the US National Bureau of Standards and the British Standards Institution. So, who was Munsell? In 1903 Albert Munsell – also an artist – invented a system of colour identification based on the responses of the human eye. In 1905 his System of Color Notation became universally recognized as the language of colour. In this, colours were identified as having three characteristics: hue, value and chroma.

The uses of this 'language' are innumerable, particularly in the building, printing and motor industries. The Munsell system is even used to codify all tints and dyes within the hairdressing industry. So if you colour your hair, you are already using the Munsell system.

All three Munsell characteristics – **hue**, **value** and **chroma** – can be referred to when describing a colour.

Hue – undertone

Hue defines a colour's undertone, which may be warm (yellow-based) or cool (blue-based). Colours such as red, pink and green can be described as having either a warm or a cool undertone. You might have a cool 'blue' red (say, a plum-coloured red) or a warm 'orange' red (a tomato red); likewise, you can have a warm olive green (yellow-based) or a cool pine green (blue-based).

Value – depth

The value of a colour refers to its depth, giving a measure of its lightness or darkness. Munsell used a scale of 0 to 10, with black being 0 and white being 10, with all the shades of grey in between. This grading of light and dark can be used to measure the depth of all other colours, too; for example, in hairdressing these numbers determine the depth of colour of a hair dye.

Chroma – clarity

Chroma indicates the purity or clarity of a colour. Some colours are bright and vibrant and reflect the light, while others are dusty or muted and seem to absorb light. The type of fabric will also determine whether light is absorbed or reflected; for example, satin reflects light while wool seems to absorb it. The chroma scale ranges from 0 to 14, with 0 being the most greyed or muted and 14 being the clearest.

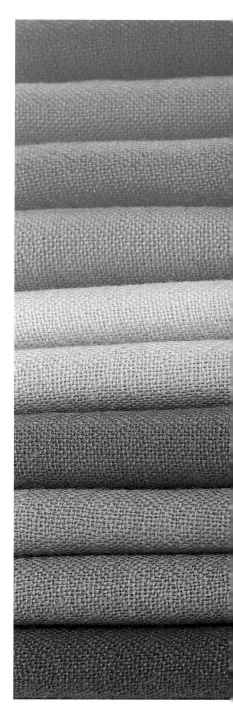

How does colour analysis work?

The process of analysis looks at the undertone (hue), depth (value) and clarity (chroma) of different colours against your skin, eyes and hair to determine your dominant type. Work through this section to discover your own colouring type.

Colour analysis was made popular by **colour me beautiful**. Millions of women have had a colour analysis with a fully trained consultant in either a studio or the workplace. When you visit a **colour me beautiful** consultant they will look at your combination of hair colour, eye colour and skin tone. This is the beginning of a process of elimination to determine which one of the six dominant colouring types you are – **Light** or **Deep**, **Warm** or **Cool**, **Clear** or **Soft**: *go to pages 34–105*.

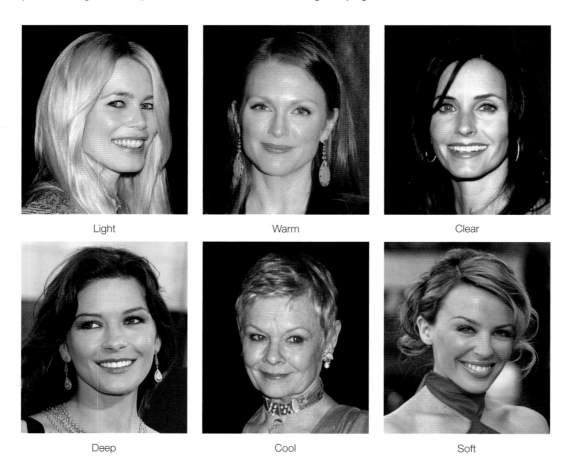

Light

Warm

Clear

Deep

Cool

Soft

The time of your life

We are all born with perfect skin, beautiful eyes and healthy hair, the colours of which are all genetically balanced together. Over the years environment, diet and everyday stresses can all take their toll on how we look. You may, for example, live in a climate where your natural hair colour becomes sun-streaked and your skin acquires an olive tone.

When the hormones start up – first in your teens and then again at the time of menopause – it's all change again. If you look at a photograph of yourself as a young child, and then as a teenager, you may well see a marked difference in hair colour. The gorgeous platinum blonde child has now become a young woman with dark blonde hair. That young woman matures gracefully into an ash-grey grandmother. In addition, of course, she may have played with nature during countless trips to a colourist at the hairdressers. Similarly, a beautiful red mane will gently fade and possibly even go grey, while the head of striking ebony hair will be the one to show early signs of white. Skin tone will have been affected by those hormones, as well as by climate, diet and lifestyle. As we age, our eye colour may also lighten and soften.

If you were colour analysed some years ago, you may well have changed in the meantime. You may now feel less happy than you were 15 years ago wearing certain recommended colours. For this reason, the idea that a person is one 'season' or palette all their life is no longer held to be true.

Elizabeth Taylor's colouring went from Clear and Warm in her youth to Soft and Cool as she reached her sixties.

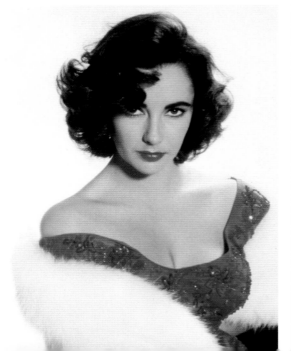

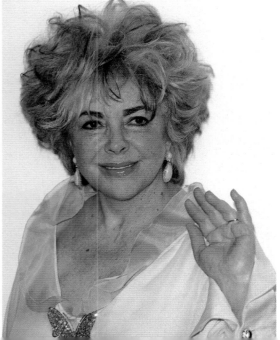

The psychology of colour

Much research has been done on the psychology of colour and its effects on everyday life. Colour can affect your mood and your energy levels profoundly, and therefore has a great impact on your general sense of wellbeing. It will also affect how others view you, from your partner to your boss.

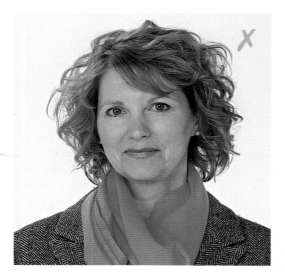

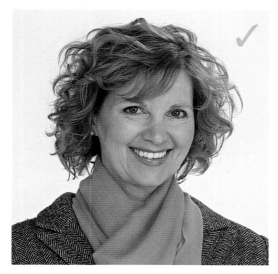

Before you get to find out about your own colouring type, let us first take a look at the psychological effect on yourself and others when you wear certain colours: *go to pages 29–31*. This is not gleaned from the results of scientific research, but from the knowledge and vast experience that **colour me beautiful** has gained over the years in the course of meeting so many women.

Investment buys

For each of the six dominant colouring types, we have suggested – and commented on – the best colours for investments buys. These are the items that you want to remain in your wardrobe for as long as possible, as opposed to the fun tops and sandals that you are happy to wear for just a few months. Investment buys are most likely to be coats, jackets and trousers; they could also be a fabulous cashmere sweater or even a handbag.

The blue undertone of the hot pink scarf casts dark shadows onto her face, while the yellow-based terracotta scarf lights up her complexion, giving her a healthy glow.

black/grey

Black can portray an air of authority and it is worn by many women as a uniform for business

Wearing black from head to toe every day is easy and safe but may give the message that you lack imagination. It also implies that you are hiding behind the colour. It might be a good idea to wear black with another colour for greater impact. For example, a little black evening dress can be a winner; if black is not in your palette, wear it with accessories near your face (pearls or beads) that tone well with your natural colouring. A pashmina or chiffon scarf in your colours will be perfect. Or, you could wear a suitable grey – either charcoal, medium grey or pewter – instead.

brown

Brown, the colour of the earth, is a great colour to wear when you're in relaxed mode

The brown family comes in many guises: chocolate, coffee, mahogany and golden, to name but a few. Brown denotes a friendly, down-to-earth, though serious, attitude. We are often told that brown is 'this season's black', and it provides an excellent alternative for those with Warm colouring, especially when you want to appear less threatening. Brown may be considered boring when worn on its own, but mixing it with other colours can bring it to life and it could become a staple of your wardrobe.

Make sure you choose the correct shade for you by checking which brown is in your dominant palette.

beige

This family of colours is a great substitute for black and browns in summer

The beiges run from stone to camel via taupe, pewter, cocoa and natural. All of these tones are non-threatening, friendly and approachable; they are excellent when you want people to open up to you. They are ideal colours for anyone who works with people, for example in counselling, human resources and nursing.

If your colouring is either Deep (pages 46–57) or Clear (pages 82–93), beige generally needs to be worn together with contrasting colours.

The joy of these tones is that they may be worn all year round with the fashion colours from your palette.

white

White denotes purity and freshness

Everyone needs white in their palette, whether worn head to toe for a special outing or as a contrast against other colours from your palette. It can be a hard colour to wear in its purest form, but there are shades of white to suit everyone, from soft white to ivory and cream; once you have identified your dominant colouring type on the following pages, refer to your colour palette to see which shade is the best for you.

Wearing white in a textured fabric will often soften its appearance. Linen and silk, for example, are rarely a pure white, although cotton can be. White is an ideal colour to wear in hot climates as it reflects light – the challenge is keeping it clean and fresh-looking.

blue

Blue, the colour of logic, activates the mind

Blue conveys trust, peace and order – it could be considered safe. When a leading British scarf retailer commissioned a survey to find out which colours sold best, blue came top. Dark navy is often associated with authority and law and order; many police forces use navy for their uniforms.

Medium shades of blue, such as cornflower, lapis and sapphire, are all great colours to brighten up your wardrobe throughout the year. The lighter shades, such as powder blue, eau de nil, bluebell and sky blue, make wonderful colours for special occasions when a feminine look may be required. Teamed with darker shades (navy and grey) they become great colours for shirts and tops.

pink

Wearing pink suggests gentleness and empathy; it brings out the femininity in every woman

All women need some pink in their wardrobe, whether it is for a dressing gown, some underwear or a pashmina. Wearing a powder pink outfit will not be your most powerful look, but a blush pink or cyclamen pink worn under a business suit will give you authority. Or, wow them on the dance floor with any shade of pink from apricot to fuchsia – but not worn head to toe.

Pink is a great colour to wear when you are feeling a little off colour, as it gives a flattering lift to any complexion.

purple

In its pure form, purple shows creativity as well as indicating sensitivity

The purple family runs from softest lavender to deepest damson. It is a great alternative – and a more exciting one – to black and navy. Beware that its creative signal does not compromise a situation where you want to appear conformist. Purple is also the colour of spiritualism and meditation. In its lighter forms, the lilacs and soft violets promote a general sense of relaxation.

Many people fight shy of purple, but if you've never worn it, give it a try in a scarf or pashmina. You'll be amazed at the effect it has on others.

red

Red is the colour of energy. Wear red and you will feel confident and in control

The red family has many variations from raspberry to tomato, so getting the undertone right is crucial. Is it warm (yellow-based) or cool (blue-based)?

Wearing red will bring excitement into your day. It is the colour of stimulation, showing a sense of exhilaration but also suggesting a demanding character. It is a great colour to wear at the end of the week when your energy level might be flagging. Do not, however, wear red when trying to calm children at bedtime.

When wearing red, take care over choosing your lipstick. Make sure it is in the same tone, although it can be lighter or darker.

green

Green, the colour of grass and leaves, conveys a sense of calm and reassurance

When wearing green, whether olive or lime, or anything in between, you show creativity and imagination. It was once thought to be unlucky, but in the world of fashion green brings another dimension to the wardrobe. With all its various shades, green may be used for virtually any garment, from a winter coat to a fun pair of shoes.

With green, it is particularly important to understand the undertone and to know whether you are better in a warm (yellow-based) green, such as moss or apple green, or the cool (blue-based) green of spruce or sea green.

Gaining colour confidence

All you need to do to work out which are the best colours for you is to follow the simple steps outlined below. These are covered in more detail in the following sections on each colouring type: Light, Deep, Warm, Cool, Soft and Clear.

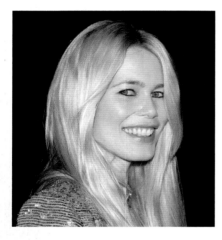

Step 1 – finding your dominant colouring

Look through the following pages and decide which of our celebrity's colouring most closely resembles yours.

✓ Do you have light hair and light eyes? **Go to page 34**.

✓ Do you have dark hair and dark eyes? **Go to page 46**.

✓ Does your hair have red tones? **Go to page 58**.

✓ Do you have grey tones to your hair? **Go to page 70**.

✓ Is your hair dark but your eyes light? **Go to page 82**.

✓ Or are you a mixture of all? **Go to page 94**.

Once you have identified the celebrity, this indicates your dominant colouring type. Read through that section (Light, Deep, Warm and so on) to understand how your 30 best colours will work for you.

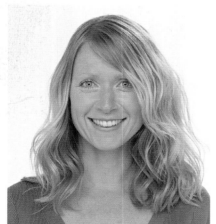

A dominant Light colouring is indicated by blonde hair and pale eyes and skin (top); golden tones to hair and skin indicate a secondary characteristic of Warm (below).

Step 2 – finding your secondary characteristic

Now see if there is a definite undertone of warm or cool to your skin. Look at the underside of your arm (which will not be sun-damaged). Warm skins have a yellow undertone, while cool skins are pinkish. The best way to see this is by doing a comparison test with your friends. Some people will show neither a warm nor cool undertone to their skin – they have a neutral skin. If you have a natural tan, this should not affect the undertone of your skin.

The colour test

Within the sections for each dominant colouring type – Light, Deep, Warm, Cool, Clear and Soft – are two sub-sections. Each sub-section suggests different colours to try against your skin in order to determine your secondary colour characteristic: *go to pages 34–105*.

Find examples of the suggested colours, using scarves, tops or any other garment that you can easily hold near your face. If necessary, borrow from your friends – you could also ask for their help in deciding which of the colours under scrutiny are best for you.

Sit in front of a mirror with no make-up on. Make sure you are in a well-lit area, with no shadows falling on your face. Natural daylight is preferable. Hold each of the suggested colours in turn under your chin and look at the result. Does the colour show on your chin? Does the colour make your complexion change?

You'll know the colour is right when:

✓ Your face appears to be lit from underneath.

✓ Your skin appears smoother, fresher and younger; lines and blemishes are minimized.

✓ Your eye colour is enhanced.

✓ You notice YOU more than the colour.

You'll identify the wrong colours when:

✗ There are dark or coloured shadows around your chin and neck.

✗ Your complexion looks uneven in colour.

✗ The colour stands out more than you.

You can now focus on your secondary characteristic, which adds 12 additional colours to your 30 dominant colours, giving 42 colours that you can use with confidence, in the knowledge that these are the right choices for you.

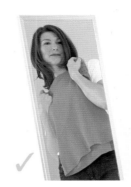
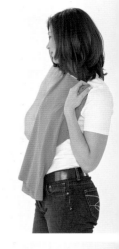
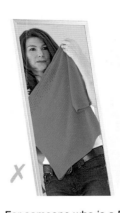
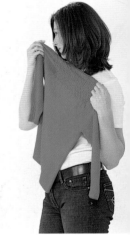

For someone who is a Deep and Warm, the colour test will reveal that salmon is a more flattering shade of pink than fuchsia.

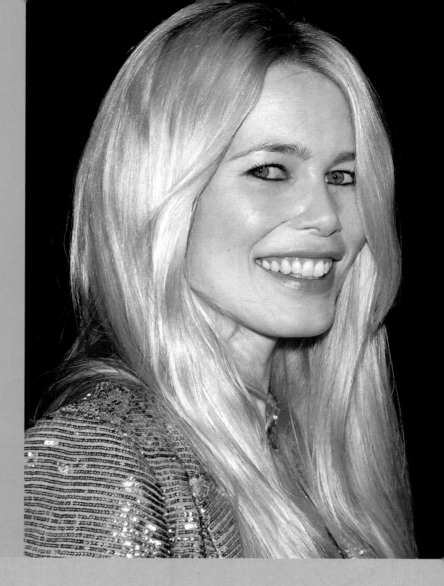

light

With her pale blonde hair, porcelain skin and blue eyes, German supermodel Claudia Schiffer is an archetypal Light.

Are you a **Light**?

Do you have

- [ ] naturally blonde or very light hair?
- [ ] pale blue, grey or light green eyes?
- [ ] pale eyelashes?
- [ ] pale or indistinguishable eyebrows which you often pencil in?
- [ ] delicate skin, probably porcelain in tone, that burns easily in the sun?

Your look is

✓ Light and delicate.

✓ The undertone of your skin may be either warm or cool.

✓ The depth of your colouring is light.

✓ The clarity of your look may be either clear or soft.

Your ideal colours

For a master colour palette: *go to pages 36–37*.

How to wear your colours

Balance your dominant look by wearing light or medium-depth colour near your face. If you have to choose a darker tone, such as light navy, for a jacket, try to contrast it with a light shade such as light apricot, rather than with a deep one like geranium.

Wear two light colours together or a combination of light and dark – but never wear two dark colours together. Always aim to have the lighter colours close to your face.

Be aware

Shopping may be a challenge in the winter season, especially when you are looking for a coat or jacket, as these are traditionally dark in colour. Try rose brown – or wear a scarf or pashmina in a light shade over your coat.

Investment buys

When it comes to buying items that you expect to keep for more than a season or two, the colours below are great substitutes for black. They do not date and you can wear them all year.

stone   taupe   cocoa   pewter

Now find out whether you are Light and Warm: *go to page 38* or Light and Cool: *go to page 42*.

Light colour palette

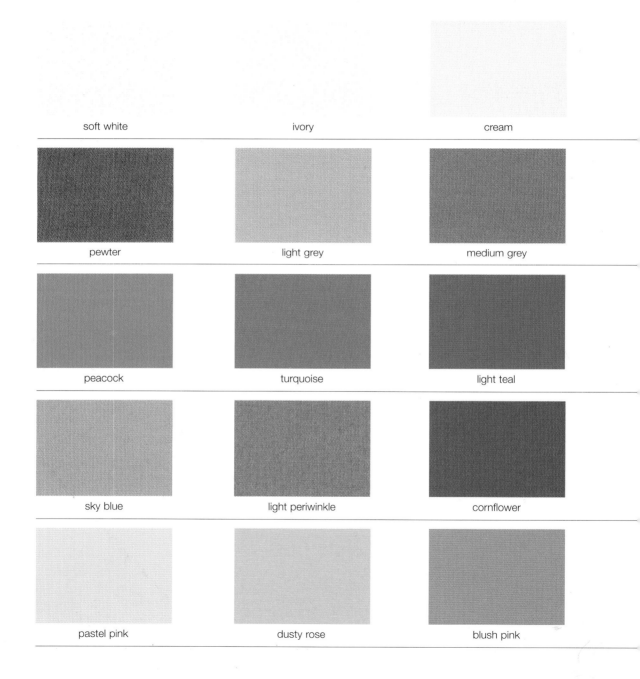

soft white   ivory   cream

pewter   light grey   medium grey

peacock   turquoise   light teal

sky blue   light periwinkle   cornflower

pastel pink   dusty rose   blush pink

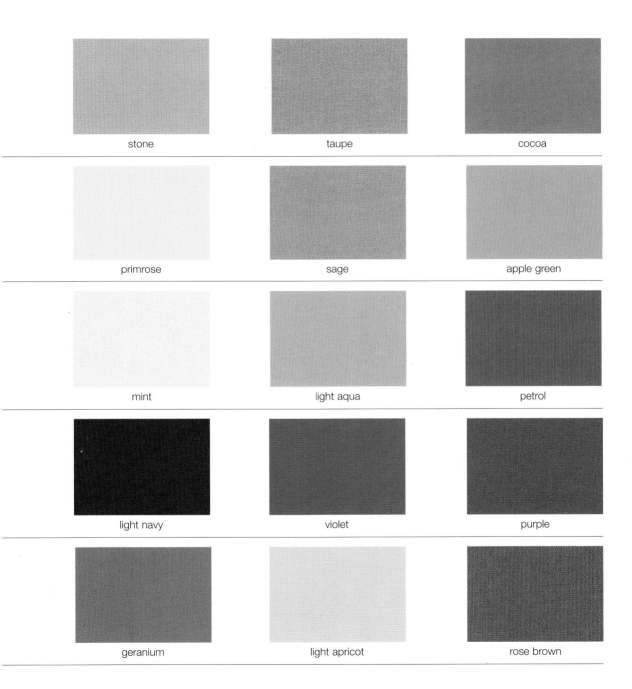

stone

taupe

cocoa

primrose

sage

apple green

mint

light aqua

petrol

light navy

violet

purple

geranium

light apricot

rose brown

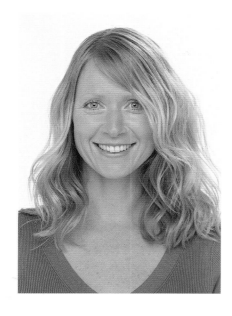

Light & warm

✓ Take a close look at your hair colour. When you are in sunlight or under a spotlight, do you see warm or strawberry-blonde tints in your hair?

✓ Does your skin have a golden tone?

✓ Do your eyes have a brightness to them?

✓ Do the colour test with peach and powder pink, and with light moss and sea green: **go to page 33**. You should find that your best pink is peach, a warm shade with yellow undertones, while the light moss will suit you better than the sea green.

Your secondary characteristic is warm. There is a clarity to your additional colours which will complement your bright eyes.

Your additional colours

As a Light and Warm, you can now add these 12 extra shades to your master palette. Notice that they all have a warm (yellow) undertone; avoid wearing icy shades and colours with a strong blue undertone. The greys and navy in your master palette are best worn with peach, yellow-green and lemon.

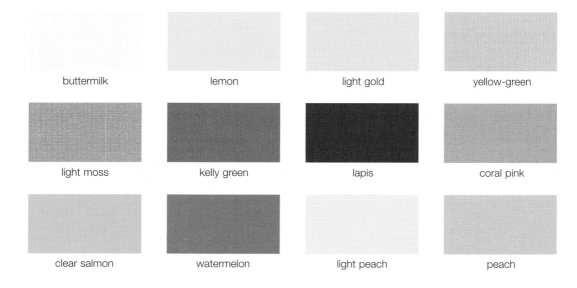

buttermilk	lemon	light gold	yellow-green
light moss	kelly green	lapis	coral pink
clear salmon	watermelon	light peach	peach

Your face

✓ The overall look of your make-up should be light and subtle. Do not overpower your delicate, warm complexion with dark, strong shades for eye shadow or lipstick.

✓ For eye pencils try coffee; you may also like teal or moss green.

✓ Accent eye shadows in light shades of green and orange, such as peppermint and toffee, will work well when blended with gold whisper or peach.

✓ Keep your blusher warm-toned, using a colour such as salmon.

✓ Lip pencils are best kept light and pale; natural is a good choice as it will not deepen your lipstick colour.

✓ Finish your look with lipstick colours such as warm pink, warm sand, coral or peachy tones, and avoid dark, muted browns.

In your make-up bag

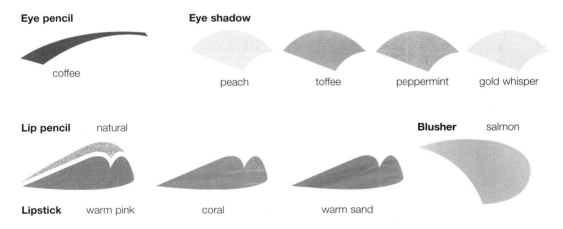

Eye pencil

coffee

Eye shadow

peach toffee peppermint gold whisper

Lip pencil natural

Lipstick warm pink coral warm sand

Blusher salmon

Your hair

✓ Of all the dominant colourings, your naturally blonde hair will need the least help through the addition of colour, though you may wish to add a few golden tones to enhance the texture; avoid the temptation to go dark.

✓ When the natural highlights that come with age start to show, go for an all-over colour that will give the appearance of golden highlights.

Mixing colours with confidence
Light & warm

Warm weather combinations

business wear

sage + light peach

light grey + light gold

taupe + yellow-green

cornflower + clear salmon

casual wear

apple green + buttermilk

light aqua + mint

light moss + pastel pink

blush pink + light periwinkle

special occasion wear

turquoise + light teal

light periwinkle + lapis

coral pink + peach

kelly green + yellow-green

Cool weather combinations

business wear

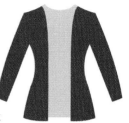

light navy + peach

rose brown + buttermilk

pewter + light moss

medium grey + coral pink

casual wear

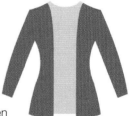

petrol + peach

watermelon + cream

light teal + lapis

cornflower + yellow-green

special occasion wear

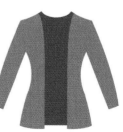

lapis + sky blue

violet + purple

geranium + coral pink

kelly green + yellow-green

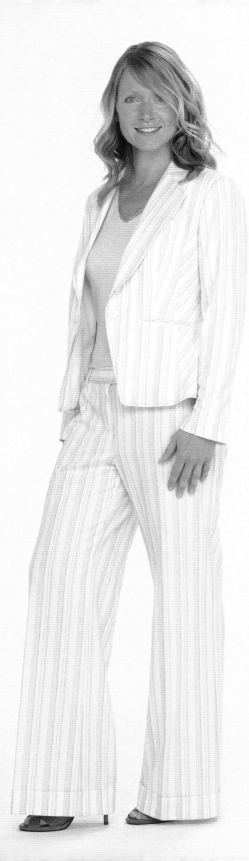

The perfect combination for someone who is Light and Warm is two light shades worn together.

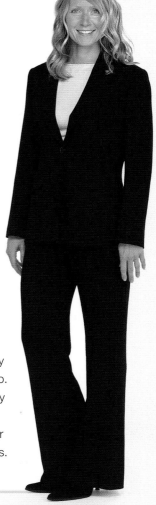

How to wear black

Black is not in your palette, but here's how to wear it for best effect. Team a black business suit with one of your light and warm colours, especially peach, light peach, yellow-green, lemon and light gold, all of which will warm up your look. Avoid the temptation to pair it with white. Don't wear black close to your face, so forgo black crew-neck T-shirts and roll-neck sweaters. For evening, try a black lacy or chiffon top. Gold or coloured jewellery will lift the black, but don't be tempted to wear stronger make-up colours.

Now that you know your colour palette, find out how to reflect your style through colour: *go to pages 138–155*.

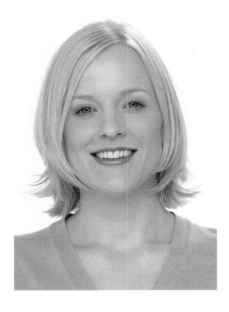

Light & cool

✓ Take a close look at your hair colour under good light. Does it have light ash tints?

✓ Does your skin have a pinkish tone?

✓ Do your eyes have a pale, misty appearance?

✓ Do the colour test with peach and powder pink, and with light moss and sea green: **go to page 33**. You should find that your best pink is powder pink, which has a cool undertone, while the sea green will suit you better than the light moss.

Your secondary characteristic is cool. Notice that there is a muted appearance to your additional colours which will complement your eyes.

Your additional colours

As a Light and Cool, you can add these 12 extra shades to your master palette; all have a cool (blue) undertone. Avoid warm shades and colours with a strong yellow undertone. Primrose or apple green from your master palette will look stunning with grey or navy.

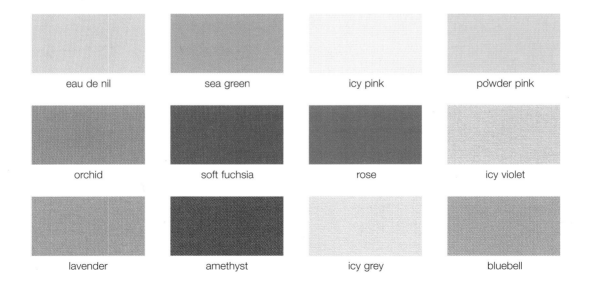

eau de nil	sea green	icy pink	powder pink
orchid	soft fuchsia	rose	icy violet
lavender	amethyst	icy grey	bluebell

Your face

✓ The overall look of your make-up should be light and subtle. Do not overpower your delicate complexion with strong, dark shades for eye shadow or lipstick.

✓ For eye pencils try granite, amethyst or dark blue.

✓ Accent eye shadows like pewter, lilac or aqua will blend well with opal or pale pink.

✓ Keep your blusher pale but make it a cool colour, such as rose or candy pink.

✓ Lip pencils are best kept light: try natural.

✓ As your colouring is light and cool, the best lipsticks will be pale soft pinks and light mauves, such as dusty rose, pink shell and bonbon; avoid coral or salmon shades.

In your make-up bag

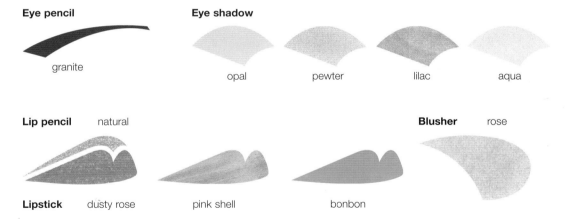

Eye pencil

granite

Eye shadow

opal   pewter   lilac   aqua

Lip pencil   natural   **Blusher**   rose

Lipstick   dusty rose   pink shell   bonbon

Your hair

✓ Your hair is naturally ash blonde, so any colour that you add to it will need to be either ash or platinum.

✓ When grey highlights start to appear as you age, they will lift the existing base tone of your hair and you will go grey beautifully – so you may prefer not to add any colour to it and let nature take its course.

✗ Avoid the temptation to add warm tones to your hair.

Mixing colours with confidence
Light & cool

Warm weather combinations

business wear

light grey + icy violet

taupe + orchid

bluebell + eau de nil

cocoa + powder pink

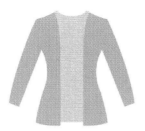

casual wear

sky blue + rose

geranium + icy grey

peacock + sea green

blush pink + icy pink

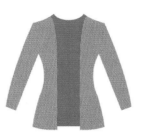

special occasion wear

lavender + violet

sea green + mint

light aqua + eau de nil

powder pink + orchid

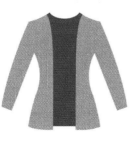

Cool weather combinations

business wear

light navy + bluebell

petrol + sea green

pewter + icy pink

medium grey + orchid

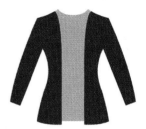

casual wear

purple + powder pink

amethyst + pastel pink

light teal + light aqua

light periwinkle + lavender

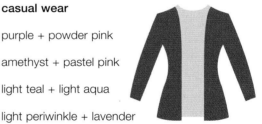

special occasion wear

amethyst + lavender

geranium + icy grey

turquoise + sea green

bluebell + light periwinkle

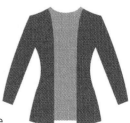

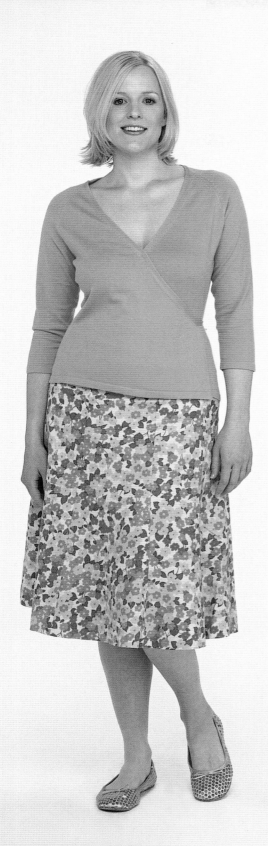

A combination of light and cool tones work best on someone who is Light and Cool.

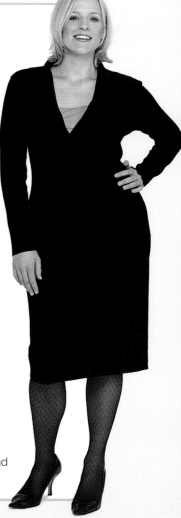

How to wear black

Black is not in your palette, but it creates a striking contrast with your ash-blonde hair. The secret is to keep black away from your face by choosing open necklines and wearing one of your key colours near your face. Softer fabrics like knits, jerseys, tweeds, corduroys and silks will absorb the light and soften the effect of the black. Your little black dress should be strappy or have a plunging neckline. Drape a chiffon scarf in one of your colours across your shoulders. Don't overpower your look by wearing a strong lipstick and heavy eye make-up.

Now that you know your colour palette, find out how to reflect your style through colour: *go to pages 138–155*.

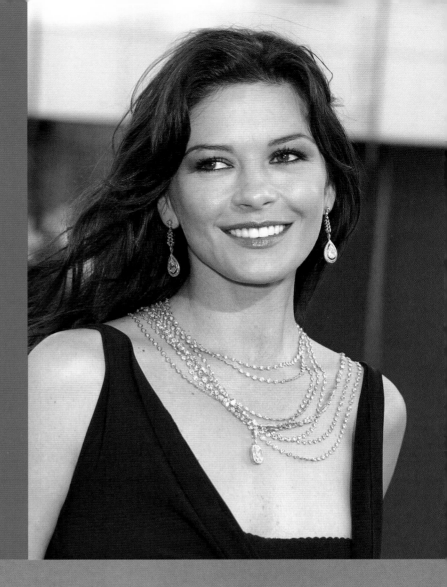

deep

With her dark hair and burnished colouring, Welsh-born actress Catherine Zeta-Jones is the perfect example of a Deep.

Are you a **Deep**?

Do you have

☐ dark brown to black hair?

☐ dark eyes?

☐ dark eyebrows and lashes?

☐ skin tone from porcelain to black, including all the shades in between?

Your look is

✓ Dark and strong.

✓ The undertone of your skin may be either warm or cool.

✓ Your overall look is deep.

✓ You may be clear or soft.

Your ideal colours

For a master colour palette: *go to pages 48–49*.

How to wear your colours

You can wear black on its own, or team it with dark shades, such as black-brown and aubergine for day or royal purple for a sophisticated look. If you are a Dramatic type (pages 146–147), try black with a single bold colour, such as scarlet.

To balance your look, wear strong, dark colours near your face. Contrast these with lighter or brighter shades from your palette. Wear two dark colours, or light and dark, but never two light colours.

Be aware

In a warmer climate you may be tempted to go for lighter shades, but be careful when wearing pale or pastel shades on their own. These will always look better on you when worn with dark or bright colours for contrast. Be bold and choose brighter colours from your palette, such as lime, emerald green, turquoise or blush pink, and combine them with stone or taupe. Remember to wear the stronger colours near your face. If you decide to wear light shades near your face, balance your look with deeper-coloured make-up so you don't look pale and washed out.

Investment buys

For the items that will have longevity in your wardrobe, choose the colours below and wear them with a darker or brighter contrast:

black	**black-brown**	**charcoal**
dark navy	**pewter**	**taupe**

Now find out whether you are Deep and Warm: *go to page 50* or Deep and Cool: *go to page 54*.

Deep colour palette

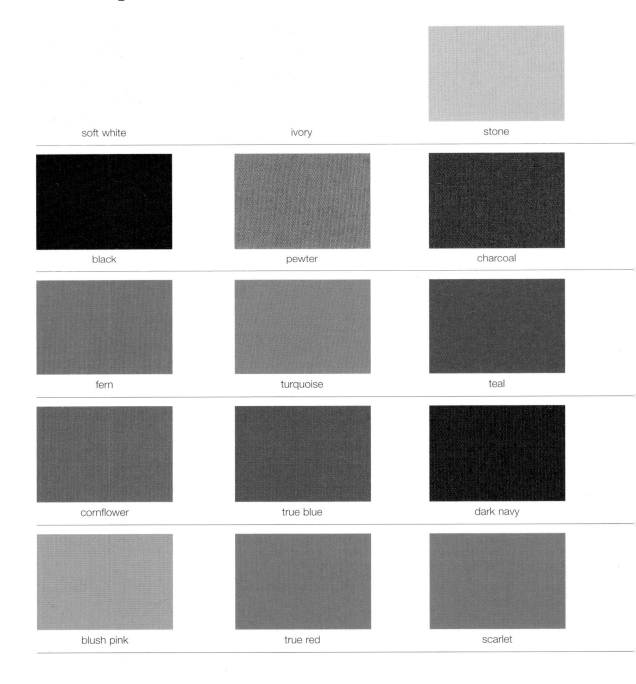

soft white	ivory	stone
black	pewter	charcoal
fern	turquoise	teal
cornflower	true blue	dark navy
blush pink	true red	scarlet

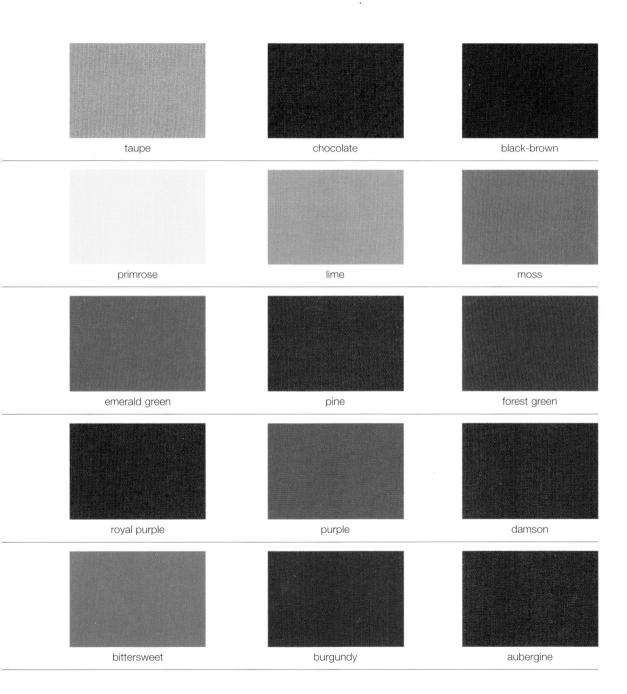

taupe	chocolate	black-brown
primrose	lime	moss
emerald green	pine	forest green
royal purple	purple	damson
bittersweet	burgundy	aubergine

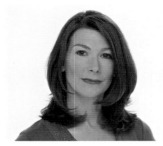

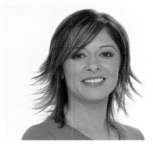

Deep & warm

✓ Take a close look at your hair colour. When in the sunlight or under a spotlight, do you see warm or red tones in your hair?

✓ Does your skin look golden and do you have some freckles?

✓ Are your eyes more golden brown than ebony brown, perhaps with flecks of green or yellow in them?

✓ Do the colour test with salmon and fuchsia, and with olive and dark teal: *go to page 33*. You should find that your best pink is salmon, a warm shade with some yellow in it, while the olive will suit you better than the dark teal.

Your secondary characteristic is warm. The softer, warmer (yellow) undertone of your additional colours will complement your look.

Your additional colours

As a Deep and Warm, you can now add these 12 extra shades to your master palette. Avoid wearing pale shades on their own and colours with an overall cool look. Charcoal, black and dark navy look best on you when warmed up with camel, salmon or terracotta.

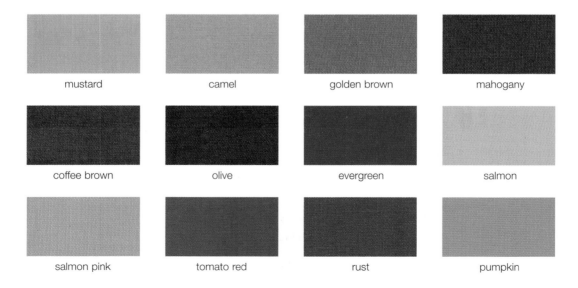

mustard	camel	golden brown	mahogany
coffee brown	olive	evergreen	salmon
salmon pink	tomato red	rust	pumpkin

Your face

✓ The overall look of your make-up should be dark and rich, with a warm undertone.

✓ For eye pencils try olive, brown or aubergine.

✓ Accent eye shadows such as khaki, smoke, mocha or other shades of brown will blend perfectly with melon, apricot or fawn.

✓ Your blusher will need some depth to it, so try rich cognac.

✓ Darker shades of lip pencil, like russet or terracotta, work best on you.

✓ Balance the richness of your complexion with lipstick shades like tomato, pecan, tamarind or terracotta; if you prefer a softer colour you will need to ensure that your eyes have a strong look for balance.

In your make-up bag

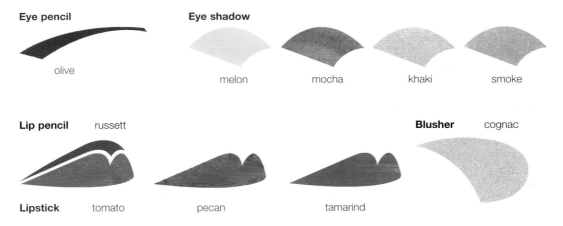

Eye pencil

olive

Eye shadow

melon   mocha   khaki   smoke

Lip pencil   russett

Blusher   cognac

Lipstick   tomato   pecan   tamarind

Your hair

✓ As your hair is dark, natural highlights – grey or white – will often start to show earlier than you expect, so don't be afraid to use permanent or semi-permanent tints.

✓ When adding colour to your hair, the key is to match the colour of your eyebrows to ensure your hair is in harmony with the rest of your look.

✓ Add red and copper tones to enhance your hair's natural warmth.

Mixing colours with confidence
Deep & warm

Warm weather combinations

business wear

coffee + mustard

golden brown + salmon

camel + tomato red

pewter + pumpkin

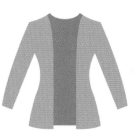

casual wear

blush pink + bittersweet

fern + rust

taupe + olive

turquoise + salmon pink

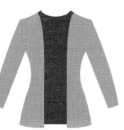

special occasion wear

lime + olive

salmon + pumpkin

mustard + primrose

tomato red + salmon pink

Cool weather combinations

business wear

aubergine + salmon

black-brown + salmon pink

pine + camel

royal purple + golden brown

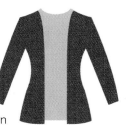

casual wear

chocolate + bittersweet

olive + scarlet

purple + camel

mahogany + moss

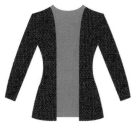

special occasion wear

true red + rust

forest + evergreen

burgundy + mahogany

damson + olive

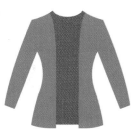

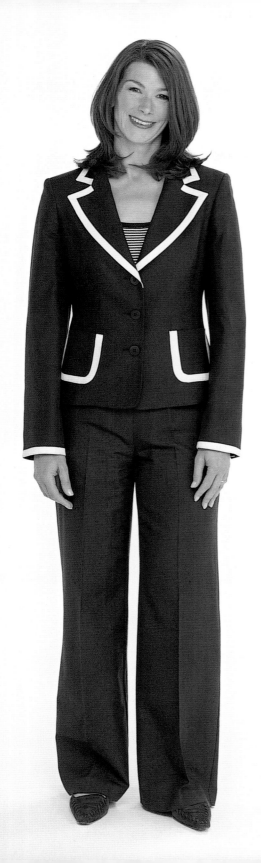

**Chocolate contrasting with ivory
is the perfect combination for
someone who is Deep and Warm.**

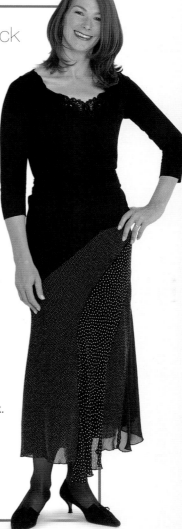

How to wear black

Black is wonderful on you
as it balances your deep,
rich colouring. Wear it as
much as you want – on
its own or with the other
colours in your deep
and warm palette. For
a stunning business
look, add tomato red or
mahogany to your black.
If you prefer, you can do
this through accessories,
with a striking red necklace
or handbag. Alternatively,
camel or coffee will work
brilliantly with black for a
softer, more approachable
look. Choose soft white
or ivory rather than a pure
white to contrast with black.
The burnished tones of the
lipsticks and blushers in
your make-up palette
enhance your overall look
when wearing black.

Now that you know your colour palette, find
out how to reflect your style through colour:
go to pages 138–155.

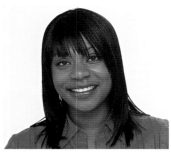

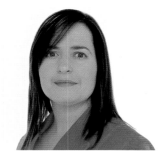

Deep & cool

✓ Take a close look at your hair colour in good light. Does it have an ebony tone?

✓ Do you have either porcelain skin or olive or black skin with a slight blue tinge?

✓ Are your eyes dark brown or ebony?

✓ Do the colour test with salmon pink and fuchsia, and with olive and teal: *go to page 33*. You should find that your best pink is the cool fuchsia, while the dark teal will suit you better than the olive.

Your secondary characteristic is cool. Notice that there is a blue undertone and a clarity to your additional colours which will complement your cool colouring.

Your additional colours

As a Deep and Cool, you can now add these 12 extra shades to your master palette. Avoid very warm shades and colours with a strong yellow undertone. When you wear lime, moss or bittersweet, balance them with royal purple, navy or pine.

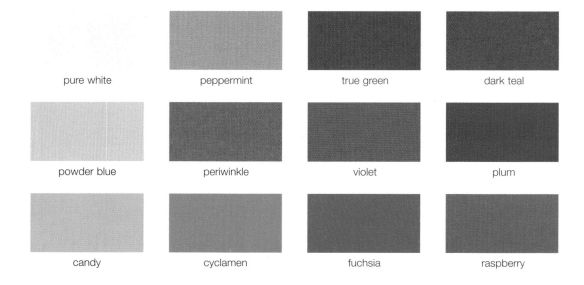

pure white	peppermint	true green	dark teal
powder blue	periwinkle	violet	plum
candy	cyclamen	fuchsia	raspberry

Your face

✓ The overall look of your make-up should be dark and rich, with a cool undertone.

✓ For eye pencils try aubergine, granite or dark blue.

✓ Accent eye shadows such as heather, blue, smoke, steel and other shades of grey will blend perfectly with pearl or pale pink.

✓ Your blusher will need some depth to it, so try cool and deep tones like port.

✓ Darker shades of lip pencil work best: try red or rose.

✓ Balance your look with bold lipsticks such as ruby, fiesta or soft mauve. If you prefer to wear a softer colour you will need to ensure that your eyes have a strong look for balance.

In your make-up bag

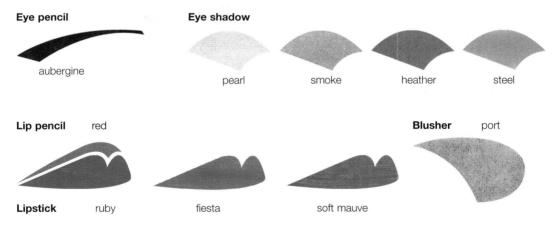

Eye pencil

aubergine

Eye shadow

pearl · smoke · heather · steel

Lip pencil red

Lipstick ruby · fiesta · soft mauve

Blusher port

Your hair

✓ Natural highlights tend to appear earlier on dark hair, but going grey will look stunning on you – though your dominant colouring may become cool.

✓ Don't be afraid to add colour using permanent or semi-permanent tints. Be guided by the natural colour of your eyebrows to make sure that your hair is in harmony with the rest of your look.

✓ Use plummy shades to enhance the cool tones of your hair; avoid red and copper.

Mixing colours with confidence
Deep & cool

Warm weather combinations

business wear

pewter + fuchsia

teal + peppermint

true blue + pure white

raspberry + ivory

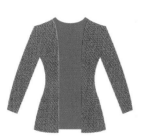

casual wear

cornflower + cyclamen

turquoise + violet

lime + true green

blush pink + raspberry

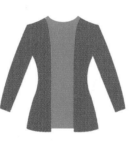

special occasion wear

peppermint + turquoise

periwinkle + royal purple

scarlet + plum

true blue + powder blue

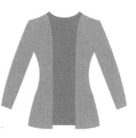

Cool weather combinations

business wear

black + chocolate

dark navy + dark teal

black-brown + plum

forest + true green

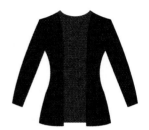

casual wear

damson + peppermint

raspberry + black

emerald green + violet

burgundy + cyclamen

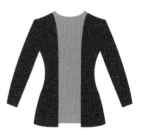

special occasion wear

true green + soft white

damson + violet

cyclamen + blush pink

black + lime

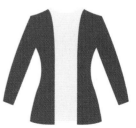

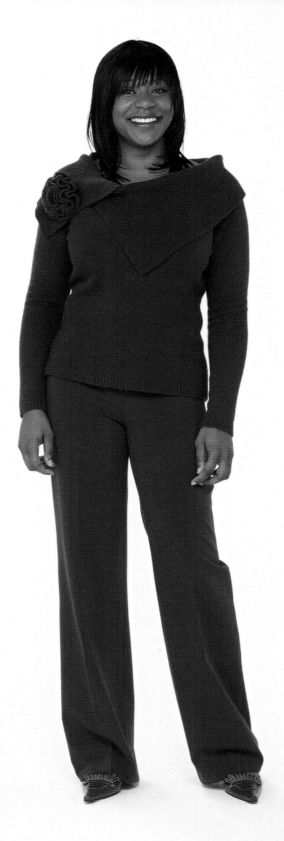

The perfect look for someone who is Deep and Cool – one dark colour worn head to toe.

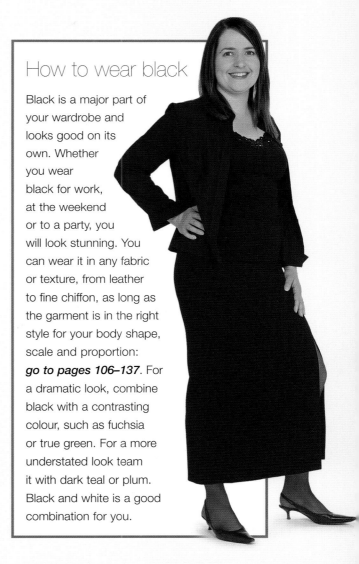

How to wear black

Black is a major part of your wardrobe and looks good on its own. Whether you wear black for work, at the weekend or to a party, you will look stunning. You can wear it in any fabric or texture, from leather to fine chiffon, as long as the garment is in the right style for your body shape, scale and proportion: *go to pages 106–137*. For a dramatic look, combine black with a contrasting colour, such as fuchsia or true green. For a more understated look team it with dark teal or plum. Black and white is a good combination for you.

Now that you know your colour palette, find out how to reflect your style through colour: *go to pages 138–155*.

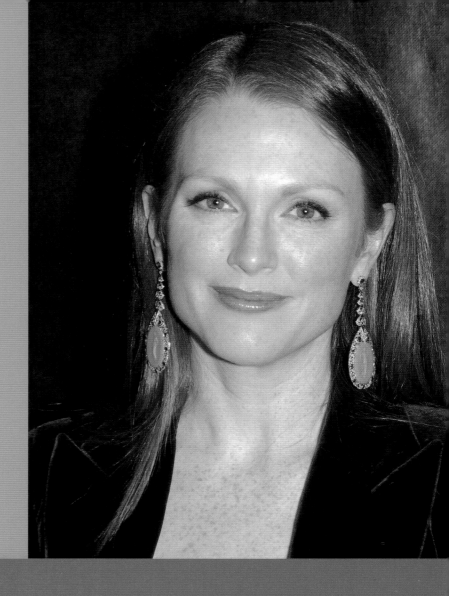

warm

American actress Julianne Moore has the russet-coloured hair and creamy porcelain skin of a classic Warm.

Are you a **Warm**?

Do you have

- [ ] red-toned hair in any shade from strawberry blonde to auburn?
- [ ] green, brown or blue eyes?
- [ ] eyebrows in a warm tone from reddish to brown?
- [ ] reddish or blonde eyelashes?
- [ ] porcelain skin, possibly with an abundance of freckles, or darker-toned skin with a golden glow to it?

Your look is

✓ Warm and golden.

✓ The undertone of your skin is warm.

✓ Your overall look is medium in depth.

✓ You may be either clear or soft.

Your ideal colours

For a master colour palette: *go to pages 60–61*.

How to wear your colours

Because your overall look is warm, the golden rule is to balance it by choosing colours that have a warm (yellow) undertone. You will always look best in colours that are medium in depth, rather than light or deep. When wearing navy or grey, warm them up with tones of yellow, salmon or peach.

Be aware

As your look is warm and golden, don't be tempted to buy items in baby pink or icy violet, as these colours will make you look grey. When wearing the darker neutrals in your palette, try to balance them with the lighter or paler shades, as your overall look should be medium in depth. Keep make-up colours warm, especially blusher and lipstick. Salmon and peachy shades will make you come alive. Avoid black mascara and eyeliner.

Investment buys

The following colours are ideal choices for items that you plan to keep for a long time. These shades will complement the majority of your other colours:

chocolate   **pewter**   **moss**

grey green   **bronze**

Now find out whether you are Warm and Soft: *go to page 62* or Warm and Clear: *go to page 66*.

Warm colour palette

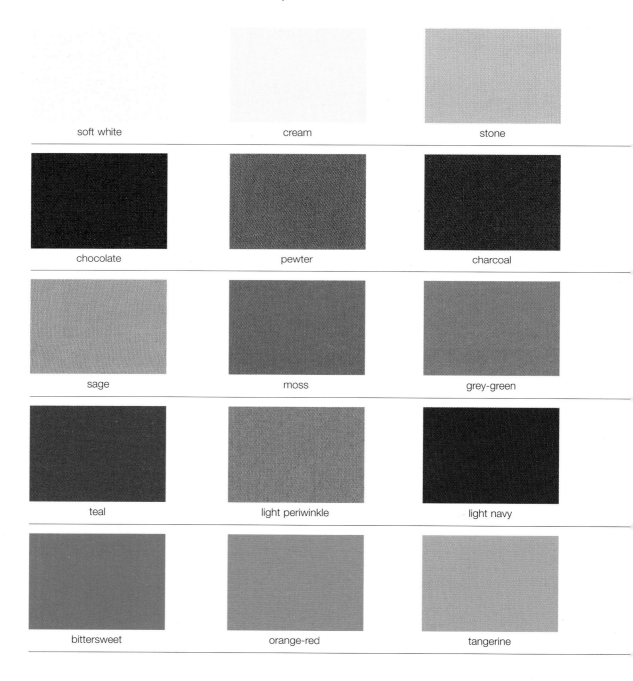

soft white	cream	stone
chocolate	pewter	charcoal
sage	moss	grey-green
teal	light periwinkle	light navy
bittersweet	orange-red	tangerine

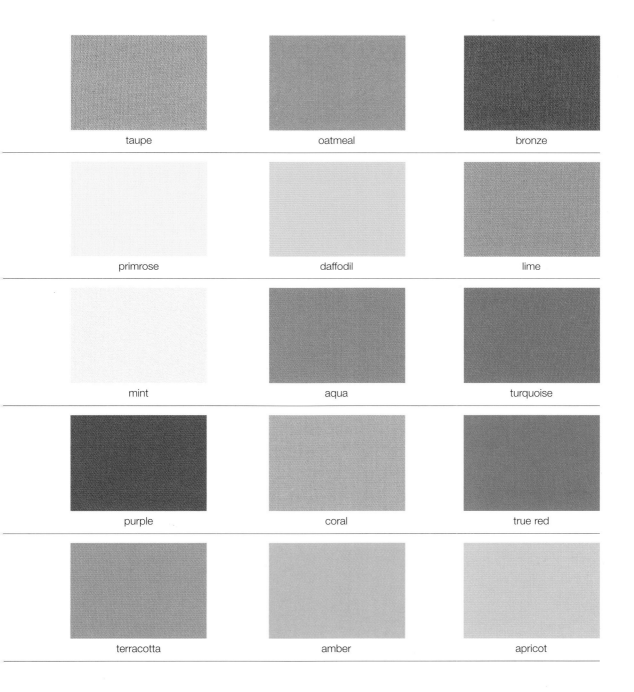

taupe	oatmeal	bronze
primrose	daffodil	lime
mint	aqua	turquoise
purple	coral	true red
terracotta	amber	apricot

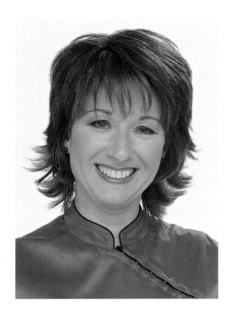

Warm & soft

✓ Take a close look at your hair colour. Would you describe it as auburn?

✓ Does your skin tone have a richness to it?

✓ Do you have brown or topaz coloured eyes?

✓ Do the colour test with pumpkin and light peach, and then with light moss and olive: ***go to page 33***. You should find that the deeper shades suit you better than the paler ones. Your best orange will be pumpkin, while the olive will suit you better than the light moss.

Your secondary characteristic is soft. Your additional colours will add depth and a softness to your main palette.

Your additional colours

As a Warm and Soft, you can now add these 12 extra shades to your master colour palette. The charcoal and light navy in your master palette can be warmed up with salmon, mustard or rust.

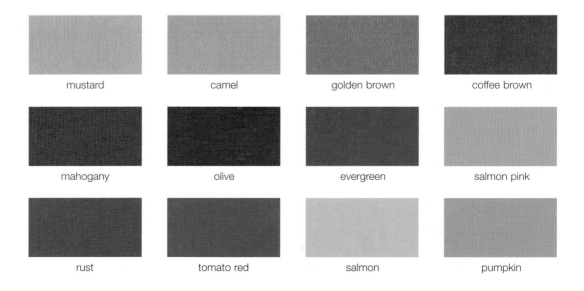

mustard	camel	golden brown	coffee brown
mahogany	olive	evergreen	salmon pink
rust	tomato red	salmon	pumpkin

Your face

✓ The overall look of your make-up should be warm and rich to enhance your golden colouring.

✓ For eye pencils try moss or brown.

✓ Accent eye shadows such as greyed green or khaki will blend well with fawn or melon, while shades of brown and tangerine will blend with apricot or toffee.

✓ Your blusher will need to be warm and golden, so try cognac or salmon.

✓ Warm shades of lip pencil work best on you: try russett or spicy browns.

✓ Balance your whole look with golden shades of lipstick such as terracotta, copper or pecan.

In your make-up bag

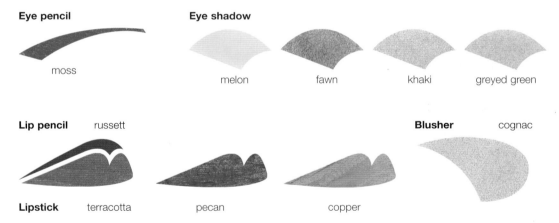

Eye pencil

moss

Eye shadow

melon   fawn   khaki   greyed green

Lip pencil   russett

Lipstick   terracotta   pecan   copper

Blusher   cognac

Your hair

✓ Your hair will be dark auburn or brown, with many warm highlights in it. Add rich warm gold or copper tones if you want to enhance the richness of the colour.

✓ When natural grey highlights start to appear, cover them with a copper or red tint; don't be tempted to go any darker or you will change your dominant colouring type.

✓ Remember, your dominant palette will also change if you leave the grey uncoloured.

Mixing colours with confidence
Warm & soft

Warm weather combinations

business wear

golden brown + coral

moss + salmon

oatmeal + tomato red

greyed green + mustard

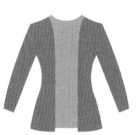

casual wear

lime + salmon pink

orange-red + rust

stone + pumpkin

light periwinkle + camel

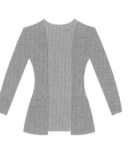

special occasion wear

tangerine + pumpkin

moss + olive

tomato red + rust

apricot + salmon pink

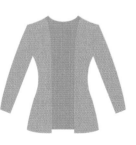

Cool weather combinations

business wear

olive + sage

chocolate + rust

charcoal + pumpkin

teal + salmon

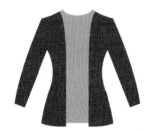

casual wear

turquoise + pumpkin

rust + amber

evergreen + lime

terracotta + coffee

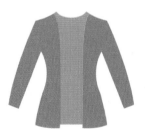

special occasion wear

coffee brown + mahogany

bittersweet + tomato red

pumpkin + tangerine

purple + mahogany

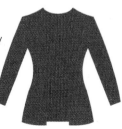

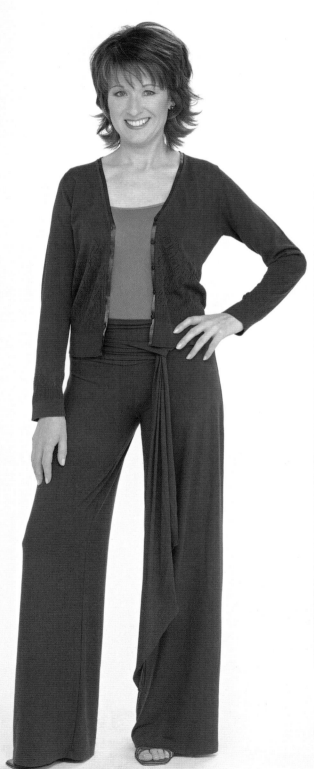

Chocolate and moss are a great colour combination for someone who is Warm and Soft.

How to wear black

Black is not in your palette and, if you have porcelain skin, wearing it near your face will make you look even paler. For best results, combine black with one of the warm and soft tones from your palette, like mustard, terracotta or salmon pink. Your little black dress needs to be soft and draping, with a low or plunging neckline to which you will need to add jewellery that will reflect warmly on your chin. Softer or textured black fabrics will be more flattering, as this type of material absorbs light, making the black appear softer.

Now that you know your colour palette, find out how to reflect your style through colour: *go to pages 138–155*.

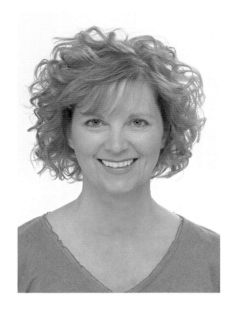

Warm & clear

✓ Take a close look at your hair colour. Is it more ginger or strawberry blonde than auburn?

✓ Do you have porcelain skin which may be sensitive to the sun?

✓ Are your eyes bright blue or green?

✓ Do the colour test with pumpkin and light peach, and then with light moss and olive: *go to page 33*. You should find that your best shades are the paler, less intense ones – light peach will suit you better than pumpkin, and the light moss will enhance your colouring more than the olive.

Your secondary characteristic is clear. Notice that your additional shades have a lightness and a clarity to them.

Your additional colours

As a Warm and Clear, you can now add these 12 extra shades to your master palette. Warm up light navy and charcoal with yellow-green, peach or light gold. Chocolate will need to be contrasted with a lighter shade like coral pink, light moss or buttermilk.

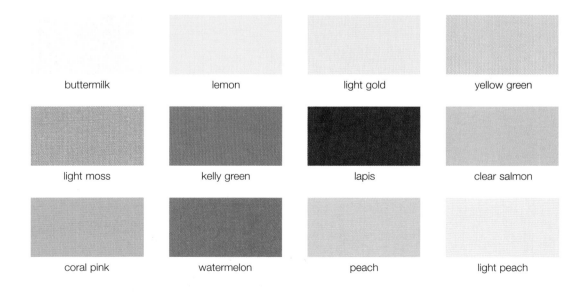

buttermilk	lemon	light gold	yellow green
light moss	kelly green	lapis	clear salmon
coral pink	watermelon	peach	light peach

Your face

✓ The overall look of your make-up should be warm, bright and clear to enhance your colouring.

✓ For eye pencils try spruce, moss green or coffee.

✓ Accent eye shadows such as peppermint or lagoon will blend perfectly with peach, toffee, shimmery gold and cream.

✓ Your blusher will need some warmth to it, so try almond or salmon.

✓ Bright, warm shades of lip pencil such as cantaloupe or coral will work best on you.

✓ Balance your whole look with lipstick in shades of coral, tulip or topaz.

In your make-up bag

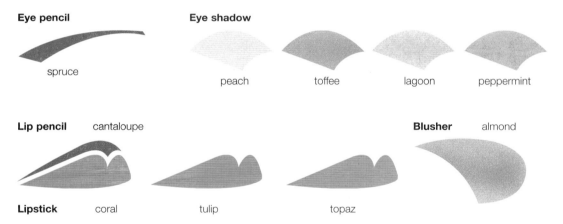

Eye pencil

spruce

Eye shadow

peach   toffee   lagoon   peppermint

Lip pencil   cantaloupe   **Blusher**   almond

Lipstick   coral   tulip   topaz

Your hair

✓ The light golden tones of your hair will naturally complement your golden skin tones, so make sure you keep your hair in peak condition to enhance the natural shine. If you want to add colour, copper or strawberry highlights will work best.

✓ Use a golden tint when the natural grey highlights start to appear. Don't be tempted to go darker or you will change your dominant colouring type.

Mixing colours with confidence
Warm & clear

Warm weather combinations

business wear

taupe + yellow-green

bronze + light peach

oatmeal + clear salmon

light navy + peach

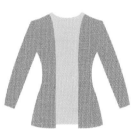

casual wear

light moss + daffodil

aqua + lapis

orange-red + peach

stone + kelly green

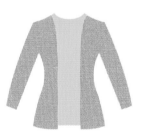

special occasion wear

periwinkle + lapis

tangerine + peach

coral pink + coral

light moss + lime

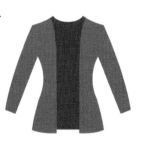

Cool weather combinations

business wear

teal + buttermilk

chocolate + peach

charcoal + coral pink

pewter + light gold

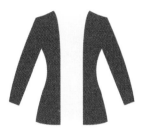

casual wear

turquoise + yellow-green

amber + light peach

true red + lapis

moss + light gold

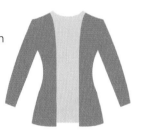

special occasion wear

terracotta + coral pink

tomato red + watermelon

purple + periwinkle

lapis + mint

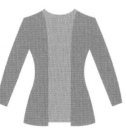

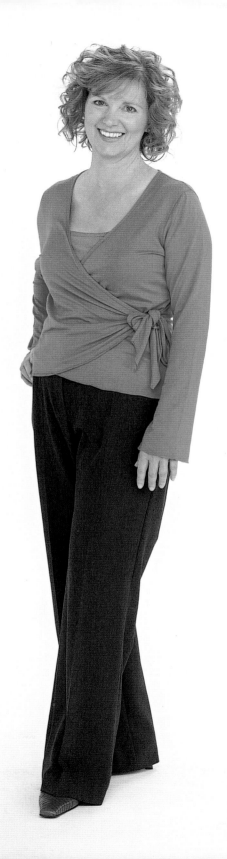

For someone who is Warm and Clear, terracotta is the perfect foil for charcoal.

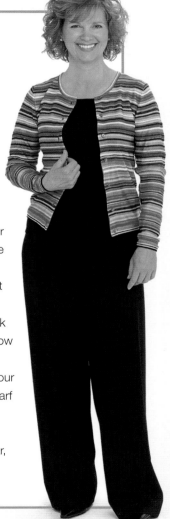

How to wear black

Black is not in your palette, but it can look striking with your brightest and clearest colours. Make sure that you have one of your best colours, such as coral pink or clear salmon, near your face. Black can also be worn with other warm or clear colours as part of a pattern or stripes. If you are wearing black on its own, choose a low neckline and add gold jewellery or beads in your colours. A coloured scarf will also help to lift the black. Keep make-up shades warm and clear, avoiding dark colours on the eyes.

Now that you know your colour palette, find out how to reflect your style through colour: *go to pages 138–155*.

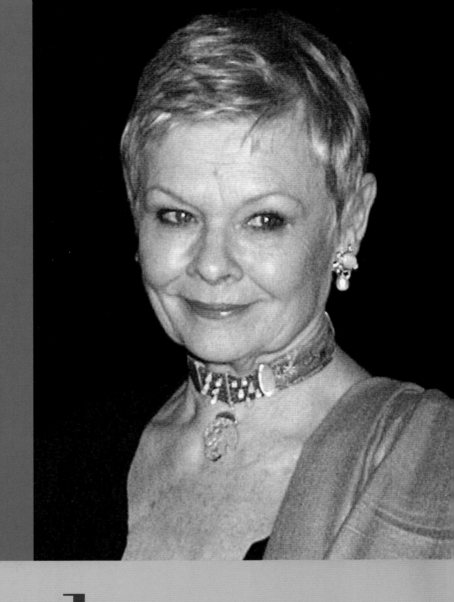

cool

Oscar-winning British actress
Judi Dench, with her distinctive
grey cropped hair, has all the
attributes of a Cool palette.

Are you a **Cool**?

Do you have

☐ ash tones to your hair, be it dark brown, blonde, white or grey?

☐ grey, blue, green or clear brown eyes?

☐ eyebrows and eyelashes that range in colour from the lighter shade of blonde to dark brown?

☐ pink undertones to your skin? A black or coloured skin may have a slight blue tinge.

Your look is

✓ Cool and pinkish.

✓ The undertone of your skin is cool.

✓ The overall depth of your colouring is medium to deep.

✓ The clarity of your look may be either clear or soft.

Your ideal colours

For a master colour palette: *go to pages 72–73*.

How to wear your colours

Because your look is cool and pinkish, all your colours need to have a cool (blue) undertone, preferably with some contrast. You will always look best in medium to deep colours. If you wear brown, balance it with cool shades from your palette, such as teal or rose pink.

Be aware

Avoid colours that have a warm, yellow tone, as these will make your skin appear sallow. If you do wear yellow, it must be an icy lemon. Browns need to have a pinky, rather than yellow, tone. When wearing your darker neutrals, balance them with the lighter and brighter shades from your colour chart and avoid wearing two dark neutrals together. Keep all your make-up colours cool and beware of brown-based lipsticks, especially pale natural-looking shades.

Investment buys

When buying items with longevity, these shades are the ideal choices and will complement most of the other colours in your cool palette:

greys   dark navy   spruce   teal

Now find out whether you are Cool and Soft: *go to page 74* or Cool and Clear: *go to page 78*.

Cool colour palette

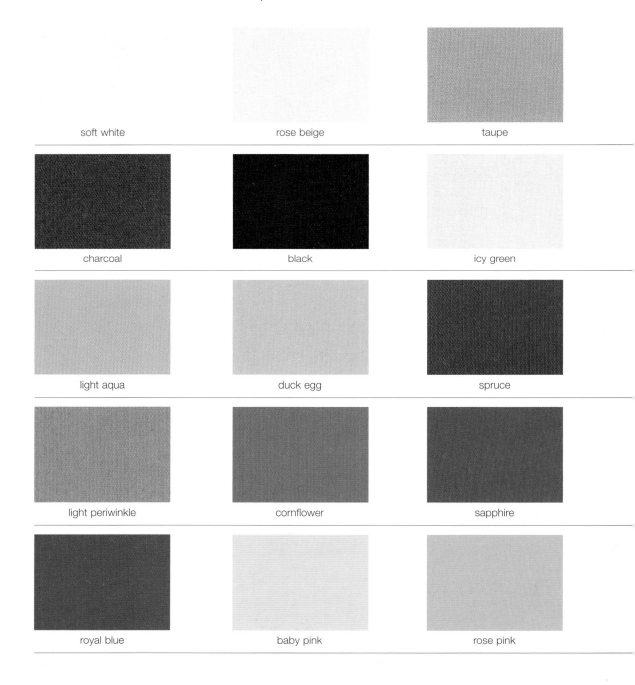

soft white	rose beige	taupe
charcoal	black	icy green
light aqua	duck egg	spruce
light periwinkle	cornflower	sapphire
royal blue	baby pink	rose pink

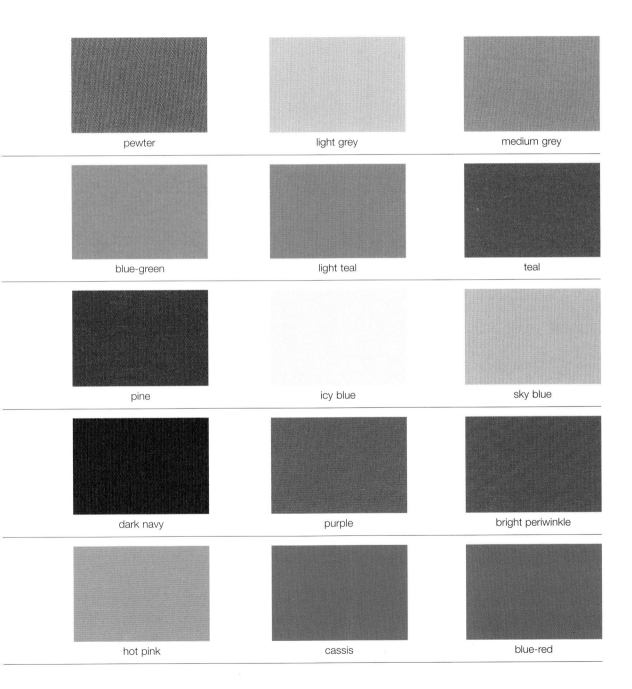

pewter

light grey

medium grey

blue-green

light teal

teal

pine

icy blue

sky blue

dark navy

purple

bright periwinkle

hot pink

cassis

blue-red

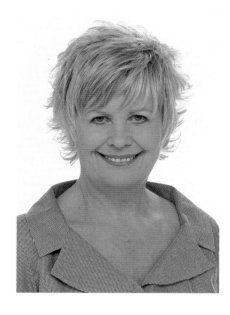

Cool & soft

✓ Take a close look at your hair colour, either in natural sunlight or under a spotlight. Does it have ash tones to it?

✓ Does your skin tone have a softness to it?

✓ Are your eyes light blue or green?

✓ Do the colour test with lavender and fuchsia, and then with amethyst and plum: **go to page 33**. You should find that you look best in the softer shades of lavender and amethyst, rather than the stronger fuchsia and plum.

Your secondary characteristic is soft. Your additional colours will add a lightness and softness to your main palette that will complement your cool colouring.

Your additional colours

As a Cool and Soft, you can now add these 12 extra shades to your master palette. When you are wearing black, soften the look by using soft pale colours, such as bluebell, powder pink or eau de nil, near your face.

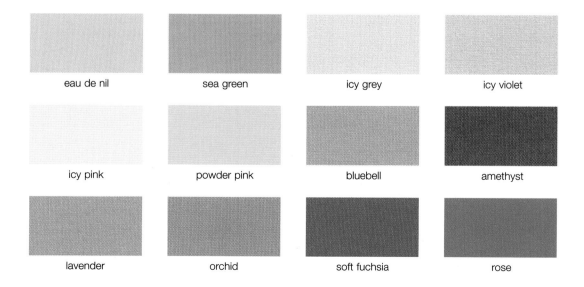

eau de nil	sea green	icy grey	icy violet
icy pink	powder pink	bluebell	amethyst
lavender	orchid	soft fuchsia	rose

Your face

✓ The overall look of your make-up should be cool, using blue-based shades to balance your dominant colouring.

✓ For eye pencils try amethyst or granite.

✓ Accent eye shadows such as heather, smoke and grey-blue shades will work well with opal, lilac or pewter greys.

✓ Your blusher will need cool pink undertones; candy or rose will suit you.

✓ Cool soft shades of lip pencil work best: try rose or pink.

✓ Balance your whole look with lipstick in all shades of cool pinks and mauves, such as bonbon, soft mauve, silk or soft berry shades.

In your make-up bag

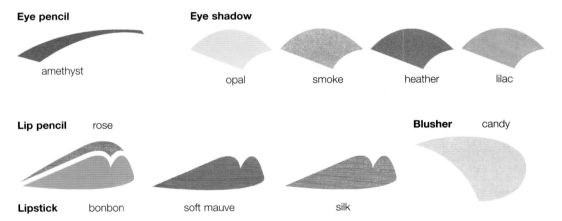

Eye pencil

amethyst

Eye shadow

opal   smoke   heather   lilac

Lip pencil   rose

Blusher   candy

Lipstick   bonbon   soft mauve   silk

Your hair

✓ Your hair will be dark blonde to light brown or a soft silvery grey.

✓ The ash tones in your hair mean that you have the advantage of greying gracefully, but you may find that you need to add a little more colour to your look by using brighter make-up or by wearing colours with more contrast.

✓ If you decide to colour your hair, make sure that you use platinum or ash tones, and avoid red tints.

Mixing colours with confidence
Cool & soft

Warm weather combinations

business wear

taupe + rose

medium grey + icy violet

sapphire + powder pink

light periwinkle + lavender

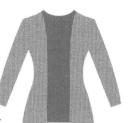

casual wear

light teal + icy pink

orchid + aqua

duck egg + icy grey

cornflower + eau de nil

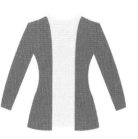

special occasion wear

sea green + blue green

amethyst + icy violet

rose pink + powder pink

bluebell + sky blue

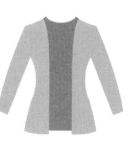

Cool weather combinations

business wear

dark navy + icy pink

charcoal + orchid

pewter + lavender

sapphire + bluebell

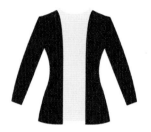

casual wear

royal blue + icy grey

rose + pastel pink

teal + soft fuchsia

purple + icy violet

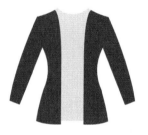

special occasion wear

cassis + soft fuchsia

blue red + rose

aqua + eau de nil

bright periwinkle + amethyst

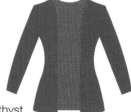

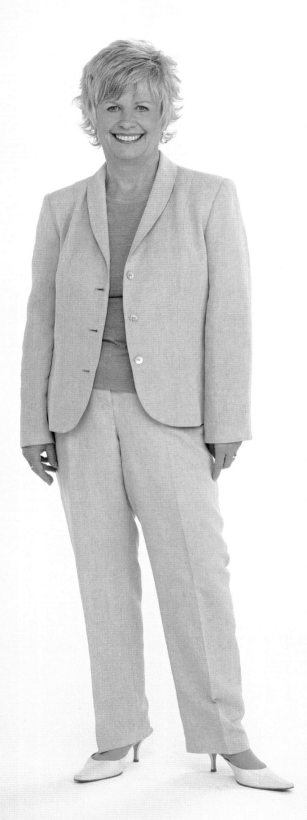

**Two contrasting shades
of turquoise make a great
combination for someone
who is Cool and Soft.**

How to wear black

Black is in your palette,
but avoid wearing it
directly under your
chin, as it may cast
a dark shadow. A
fabric with a soft
texture and weave,
such as tweed,
velvet, washed silk
or black denim, will
absorb the light,
making the black
appear less harsh. If
you wear a solid black
fabric with little texture,
add colours such as
lavender, amethyst or
powder pink near
your face to soften
the look. Your little
black dress should
be lacy or have a
low neckline. Wear
it with pearls.

Now that you know your colour palette, find
out how to reflect your style through colour:
go to pages 138–155.

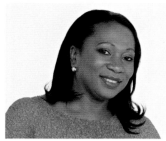

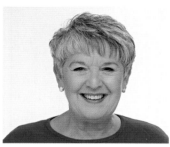

Cool & clear

✓ Take a close look at your hair colour under the light. If it is grey, is your hair more silver than ash? If you are dark-haired, is your hair really dark?

✓ Is there a clarity about your skin colour?

✓ Are your eyes dark blue, green or clear brown?

✓ Do the colour test with lavender and fuchsia, and then with amethyst and plum: *go to page 33*. You should find that you look best in fuchsia and plum.

Your secondary characteristic is clear. Your additional colours include darker shades and they will all add clarity to your main colour palette.

Your additional colours

As a Cool and Clear, you can now add these 12 extra shades to your main palette. When you wear taupe, pewter or medium to light grey, balance these lighter tones with clearer and deeper shades from your palette, such as violet, true green or raspberry.

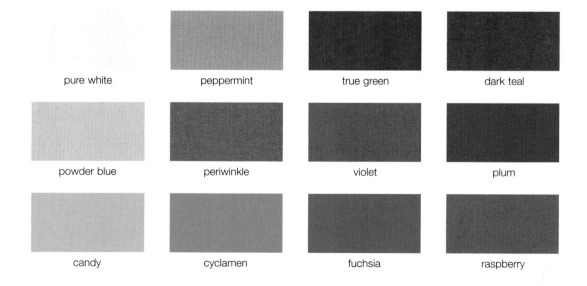

pure white	peppermint	true green	dark teal
powder blue	periwinkle	violet	plum
candy	cyclamen	fuchsia	raspberry

Your face

✓ The overall look of your make-up should be cool, using cool shades to balance your dominant colouring.

✓ For eye pencils try marine, soft black or violet-blue.

✓ Accent eye shadows such as cocoa, delph and shades of dark smoky greys will blend well with pearl, dusk or aqua.

✓ Your blusher will need to be cool, so try a shade like port.

✓ Cool shades of lip pencil like posie work best for you.

✓ Balance your whole look with cool, clear lipstick colours like cerise, fiesta or ruby.

In your make-up bag

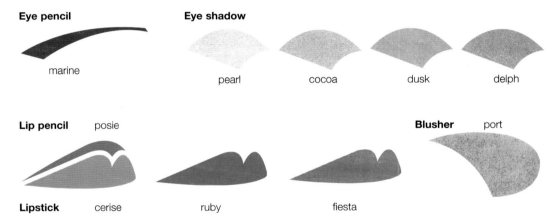

Eye pencil

marine

Eye shadow

pearl   cocoa   dusk   delph

Lip pencil   posie

Blusher   port

Lipstick   cerise   ruby   fiesta

Your hair

✓ You have dark brown or even black hair, with no apparent warmth to it. The strong colours in your palette work wonderfully with the striking cool tones of your hair.

✓ Use contrast in your make-up and clothes to balance your hair colour.

✓ When your hair eventually turns grey, it will be a stunning pure white or silver grey.

Mixing colours with confidence
Cool & clear

Warm weather combinations

business wear

pewter + fuchsia

charcoal + duck egg

periwinkle + icy blue

raspberry + pastel pink

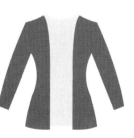

casual wear

true green + icy green

royal blue + powder blue

violet + cassis

aqua + dark teal

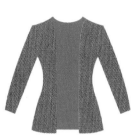

special occasion wear

cyclamen + cassis

raspberry + plum

peppermint + spruce

light grey + black

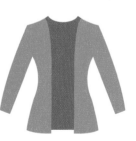

Cool weather combinations

business wear

black + powder blue

pine + peppermint

dark navy + true green

blue-red + pure white

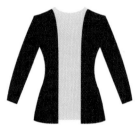

casual wear

purple + fuchsia

raspberry + spruce

periwinkle + icy blue

charcoal + cyclamen

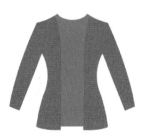

special occasion wear

dark teal + light teal

plum + cyclamen

royal blue + powder blue

black + pure white

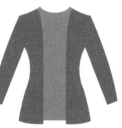

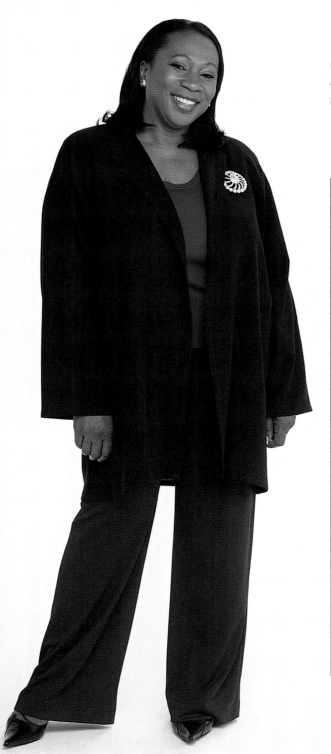

Damson and violet is a perfect combination for someone who is Cool and Clear.

How to wear black

Black is a key colour in your palette. You may wear it with many other colours as long as there is contrast, so pair black with light or bright colours, such as white, cyclamen, icy pink or fuchsia. When wearing black in a soft fabric that absorbs the light, such as tweed, velvet or knit, combine it with the darker, brighter colours of your palette, such as periwinkle, true green or raspberry. Brighten up a black jacket or top with a sparkling brooch or a stunning scarf.

Now that you know your colour palette, find out how to reflect your style through colour: *go to pages 138–155*.

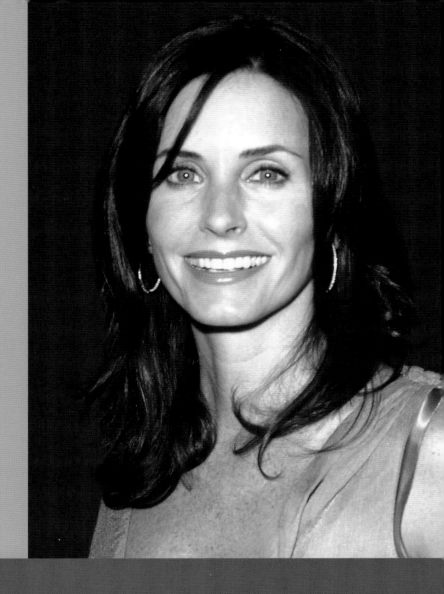

clear

Star of the TV series *Friends*, American actress Courtney Cox Arquette is a perfect example of someone classified as a Clear.

Are you a **Clear**?

Do you have

☐ dark hair?

☐ bright eyes that are your most striking feature, be they blue, green or topaz? If you are dark-skinned there will be noticeable contrast between the white of your eyes and the colour of the iris.

☐ dark eyebrows and eyelashes?

☐ skin that can be any tone from light to dark.

Your look is

✓ Fresh and clear.

✓ The undertone of your skin may be either warm or cool.

✓ Your overall look is contrasting between light and dark.

✓ You have a decidedly clear look.

Your ideal colours

For a master colour palette: *go to pages 84–85*.

How to wear your colours

Because your look is contrasting (for example, dark hair, bright eyes and, if Caucasian, porcelain skin) you need to wear your colours in a way that balances this. You will always look good in a contrast of light and dark colours. If you wear sludgy colours like taupe and pewter, liven them up with the brightest shades from your palette. If you dress in a single colour, make sure it is one of the most vivid from your palette.

Be aware

Basic neutrals like black, charcoal and chocolate are great staples in your wardrobe, but do wear them with the lighter shades from your palette. You may be tempted to wear white in summer, but combine it with a bright colour like scarlet, or even black, to keep a light and dark contrast.

Investment buys

For you, the best colours for items that will have longevity in your wardrobe are:

black	**black-brown**	**dark navy**
charcoal	**purple**	**royal blue**

Now find out whether you are Clear and Warm: *go to page 86* or Clear and Cool: *go to page 90*.

Clear colour palette

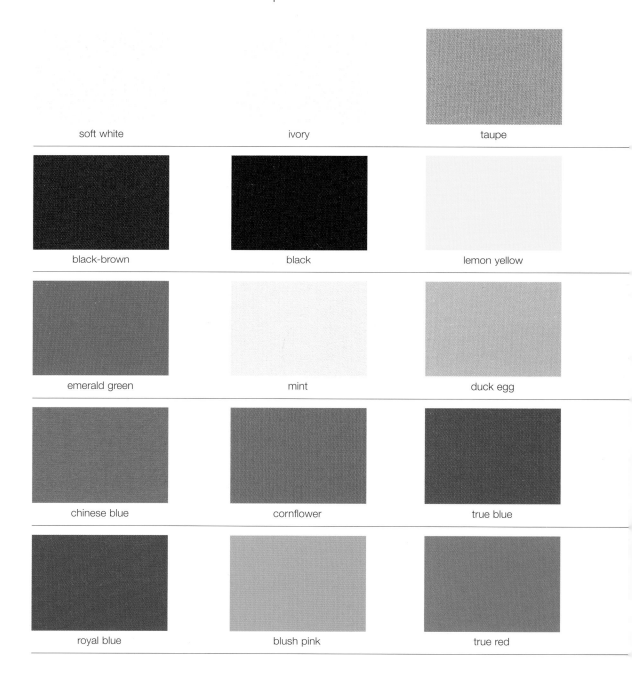

soft white	ivory	taupe
black-brown	black	lemon yellow
emerald green	mint	duck egg
chinese blue	cornflower	true blue
royal blue	blush pink	true red

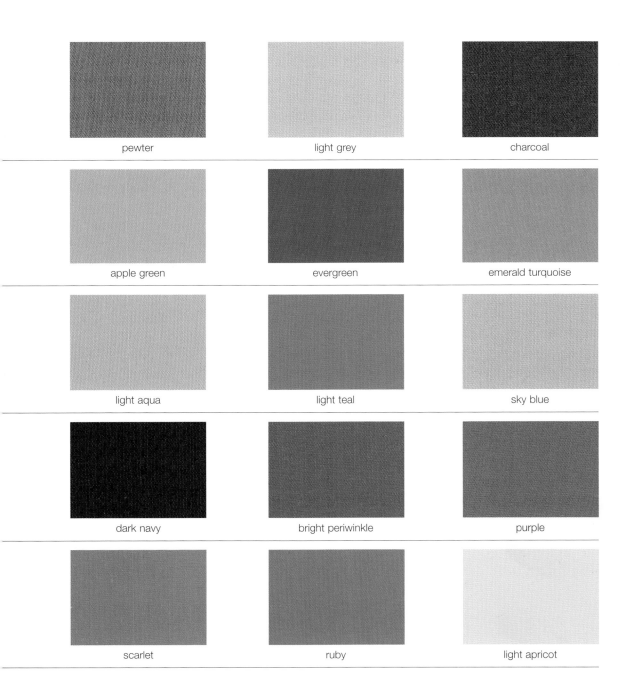

pewter

light grey

charcoal

apple green

evergreen

emerald turquoise

light aqua

light teal

sky blue

dark navy

bright periwinkle

purple

scarlet

ruby

light apricot

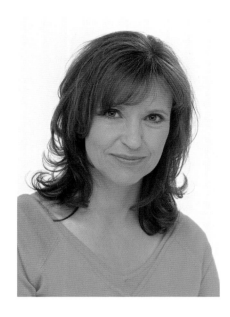

Clear & warm

✓ Take a close look at your hair colour under good light. Is it dark with warm highlights?

✓ Does your skin have warm golden undertones and maybe a few freckles?

✓ Are your eyes clear bright blue, clear green or clear topaz?

✓ Do the colour test with clear salmon and cyclamen, and then with kelly green and dark teal: *go to page 33*. You should find that your best shade of pink is a clear salmon, while the kelly green will suit you better than the dark teal.

Your secondary characteristic is warm. Your additional colours all have warmth to them and include some lighter shades.

Your additional colours

As a Clear and Warm you can add these 12 extra shades to your master palette. When you wear lighter tones, like taupe, pewter or medium to light grey, balance them with clearer, deeper shades from your palette, such as coral pink, kelly green or lapis.

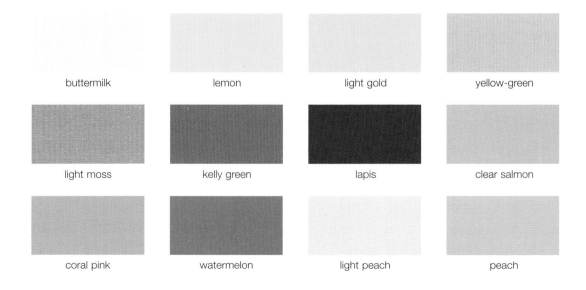

buttermilk	lemon	light gold	yellow-green
light moss	kelly green	lapis	clear salmon
coral pink	watermelon	light peach	peach

Your face

✓ The overall look of your make-up should be clear, and your contrasting look needs to be balanced with brighter colours. You may want to decide whether to emphasize either your eyes or your lips, but not both at once.

✓ For eye pencils try spruce, amethyst, violet-blue or teal.

✓ Accent eye shadows like cocoa, steel, peppermint or heather work well with melon, peach or apricot.

✓ Your blusher will need some warmth to it, so a shade such as salmon is ideal.

✓ Brighter shades of lip pencil work best: try cantaloupe.

✓ Balance your whole look with lipstick colours such as warm pink, coral or breeze.

In your make-up bag

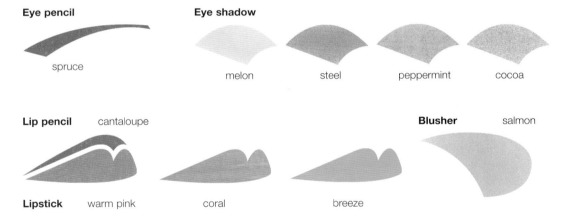

Eye pencil

spruce

Eye shadow

melon   steel   peppermint   cocoa

Lip pencil   cantaloupe

Blusher   salmon

Lipstick   warm pink   coral   breeze

Your hair

✓ Your hair will be dark but with some golden or copper highlights in it. Keep the base colour of your hair dark; don't be tempted to go blonde.

✓ If you want to add colour, it is best to use varying colours of lowlights – two to three shades will enhance your natural colour.

✓ Cover grey with a warm tint that will give the appearance of highlights. Gold or copper lowlights work well, as do warm semi-permanent tints.

Mixing colours with confidence
Clear & warm

Warm weather combinations

business wear

pewter + yellow-green

sky blue + lapis

cornflower + light gold

emerald turquoise + light peach

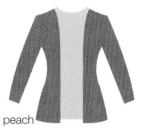

casual wear

blush pink + coral pink

taupe + watermelon

true blue + buttermilk

apple green + yellow-green

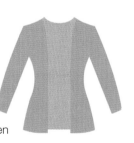

special occasion wear

light teal + buttermilk

chinese blue + mint

coral pink + light apricot

light periwinkle + light moss

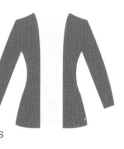

Cool weather combinations

business wear

lapis + ivory

black + clear salmon

charcoal + lemon

watermelon + light grey

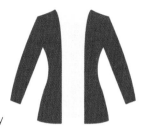

casual wear

evergreen + yellow-green

purple + coral pink

royal blue + peach

black-brown + watermelon

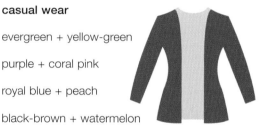

special occasion wear

cornflower + lapis

light aqua + chinese blue

ruby + clear salmon

emerald green + light moss

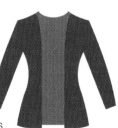

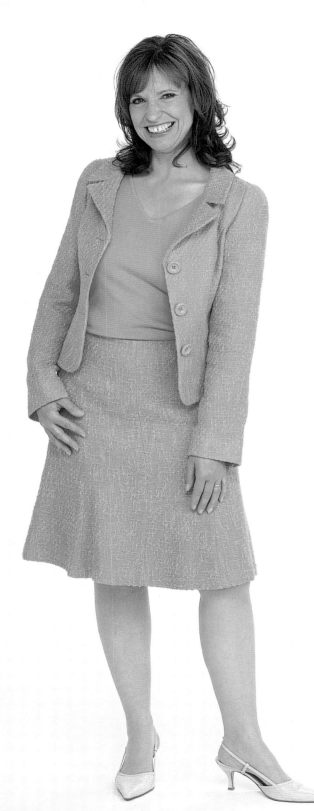

Those with a Clear and Warm colouring will look wonderful in a clear, bright colour worn head to toe.

How to wear black

Black is one of the main colours in your palette and will look stunning with a bright contrasting colour such as clear salmon, coral pink or watermelon. You may also wear it with a light colour such as lemon or light peach, but don't wear it head to toe. Complete your look with either bright eye make-up or a bright or shimmering lipstick in bright, warm and contrasting colours. For evening, accessorize black with brightly coloured jewellery or with glitter and sparkle. Alternatively, choose shiny fabrics like silk or satin which will reflect the light and look iridescent.

Now that you know your colour palette, find out how to reflect your style through colour: *go to pages 138–155*.

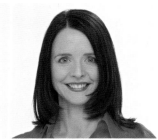

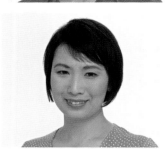

Clear & cool

✓ Take a close look at your hair colour in sunlight or under a spotlight. Does it have ebony tones?

✓ Does your porcelain skin have a pink tone to it? If you are black, does your skin have a coolness to it?

✓ Are your eyes dark green, blue or clear brown?

✓ Do the colour test with clear salmon and cyclamen, and then with kelly green and dark teal: *go to page 33*. You should find that your best shade of pink is cyclamen, while the dark teal will suit you better than the kelly green.

Your secondary characteristic is cool. Your additional colours will add coolness and depth to your main colour palette.

Your additional colours

As a Clear and Cool, you can now add these 12 extra shades to your master palette. When wearing the lighter shades of your palette, such as stone and light grey, contrast them with ruby, bright periwinkle, emerald and turquoise.

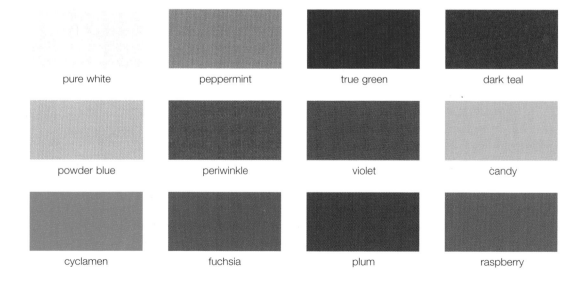

pure white	peppermint	true green	dark teal
powder blue	periwinkle	violet	candy
cyclamen	fuchsia	plum	raspberry

Your face

✓ The overall look of your make-up should be clear, and your contrasting look needs to be balanced with deeper colours.

✓ For eye pencils try petrol, dark blue or soft black.

✓ Accent eye shadows such as mercury, pewter or mocha blended with champagne or smoky greys will look wonderful on you.

✓ Your blusher needs to be cool and deep so try shades like marsala.

✓ Darker shades of lip pencil like red or bright pink work best.

✓ Balance your whole look with lipstick colours such as strawberry, ruby, fiesta or bright reds.

In your make-up bag

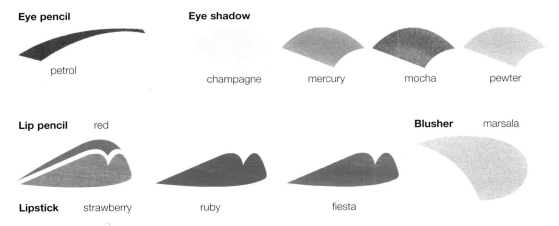

Eye pencil

petrol

Eye shadow

champagne   mercury   mocha   pewter

Lip pencil   red

Blusher   marsala

Lipstick   strawberry   ruby   fiesta

Your hair

✓ Your hair is dark brown or even black, and there will be a lack of warmth to it. If you have a dark or oriental complexion, your hair may have a slight blue tinge.

✓ When adding colour use plummy (bluish) shades and avoid copper or red tones.

✓ When natural grey highlights start to appear, cover the whole with a cool plummy tint. If you decide to go with the grey, your basic palette may change to Cool and Clear (pages 78–81).

Mixing colours with confidence
Clear & cool

Warm weather combinations

business wear

pewter + cyclamen

true blue + powder blue

true red + pure white

peppermint + dark navy

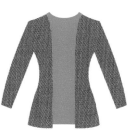

casual wear

periwinkle + light apricot

apple green + true green

scarlet + violet

dark teal + lemon yellow

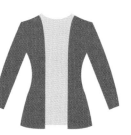

special occasion wear

chinese blue + powder blue

violet + periwinkle

peppermint + mint

blush pink + raspberry

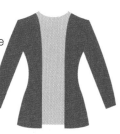

Cool weather combinations

business wear

black + ruby

true green + peppermint

navy + cyclamen

black-brown + violet

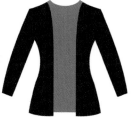

casual wear

royal blue + fuchsia

bright periwinkle + violet

charcoal + cyclamen

blush pink + plum

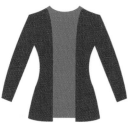

special occasion wear

evergreen + peppermint

dark teal + dark aqua

black + fuchsia

scarlet + violet

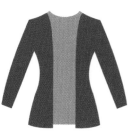

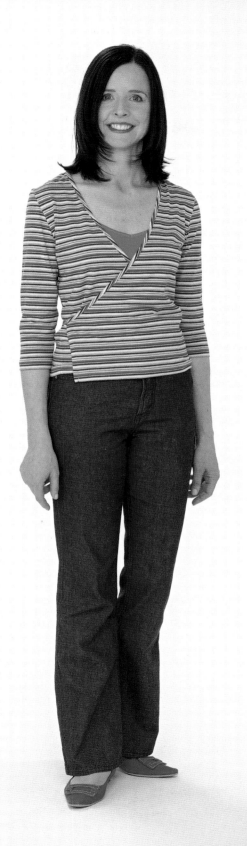

Bright and cool colours worn together work well for those who are Clear and Cool.

How to wear black

Black looks striking against the strong, dark tones of your hair and sparkling eyes. Black and pure white is a stunning combination for day and night, for any occasion. You can also combine black with pale shades, such as powder blue, striking ones, such as cyclamen, or rich colours, such as true green. When wearing black, add sheen to your eye make-up and a shimmer or gloss to your already vibrant lip colour. White gold or platinum jewellery will add lightness to black if worn on its own for evening.

Now that you know your colour palette, find out how to reflect your style through colour: *go to pages 138–155*.

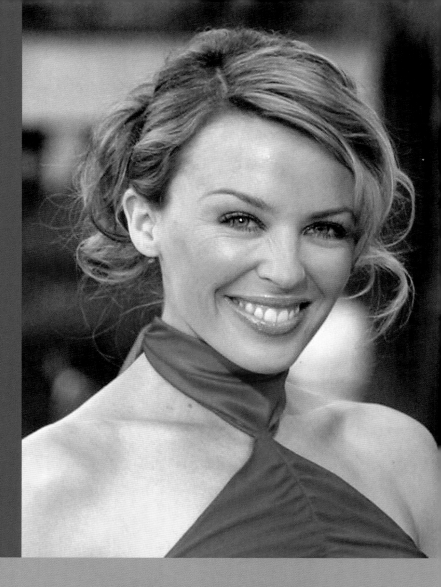

soft

With her highlighted hair
and soft skin tone, Australian
singer Kylie Minogue would
be classified as a Soft.

Are you a **Soft**?

Do you have

☐ dark blonde (mousey) or light brown hair?

☐ eyes that are a soft and muted colour, whether blue, brown, hazel or green, and that often change colour?

☐ light to dark eyebrows and eyelashes?

☐ little contrast between the colour of your hair, your eyes and your skin, which may be any tone from light to dark?

Your look is

✓ Soft, with colouring characteristics that are apparently unrelated and may be confusing. You may have found a little of yourself in each of the previous five dominant colouring types, but you do not fit any of them exactly.

✓ The undertone of your skin may be either warm or cool.

✓ The overall depth of your colouring is medium.

✓ Your look is decidedly soft.

Your ideal colours

For a master colour palette: *go to pages 96–97*.

How to wear your colours

Because your look is blended, your colours need to be worn 'tone on tone', with little contrast. You will always look best in tones of medium depth.

A monochromatic look suits you very well. If you wear the darker shades in your palette, balance them with colours that are only one or two tones lighter and avoid high contrast.

Be aware

If you like to wear strong bright colours, choose interesting combinations, like sapphire and mint, purple and geranium, or damson and blush pink. Wear pale shades like soft white or shell with medium depth colours rather than dark shades.

Investment buys

For you, the best colours for items that will have longevity in your wardrobe are:

charcoal	light navy	pewter
rose brown	taupe	stone

Now find out whether you are Soft and Warm: *go to page 98* or a Soft and Cool: *go to page 102*.

Soft colour palette

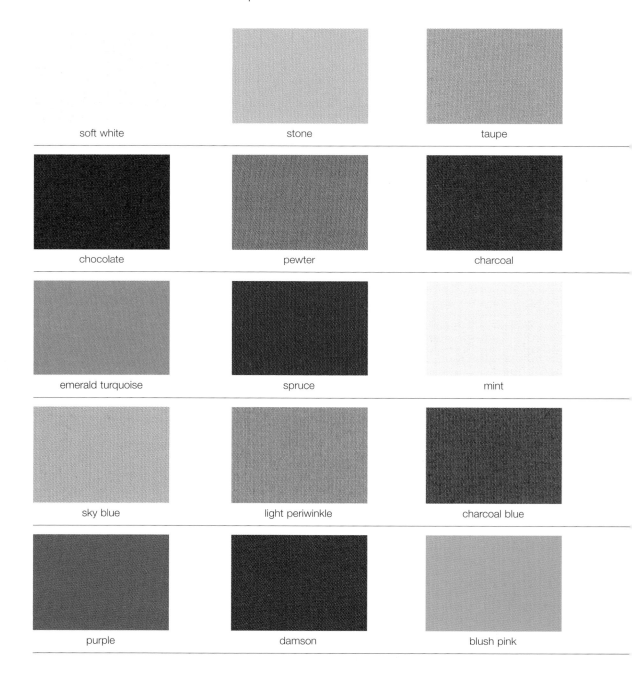

soft white	stone	taupe
chocolate	pewter	charcoal
emerald turquoise	spruce	mint
sky blue	light periwinkle	charcoal blue
purple	damson	blush pink

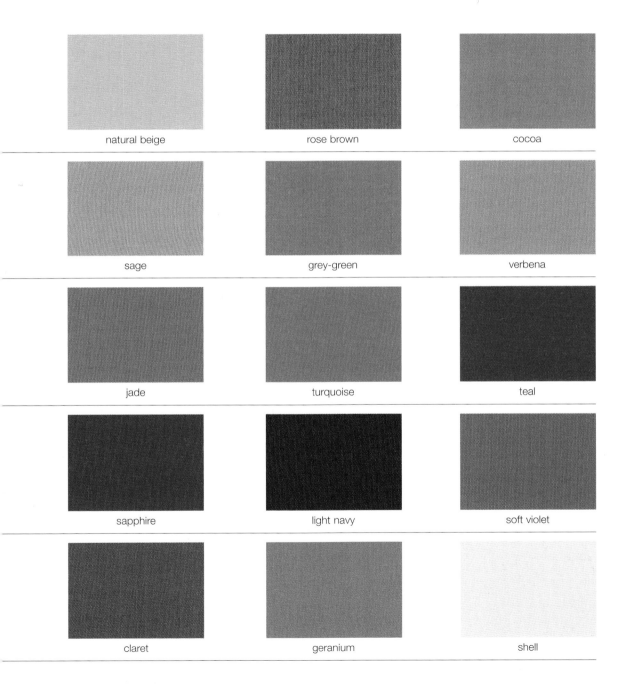

natural beige

rose brown

cocoa

sage

grey-green

verbena

jade

turquoise

teal

sapphire

light navy

soft violet

claret

geranium

shell

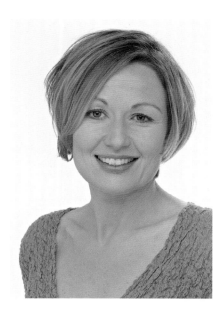

Soft & warm

✓ Take a close look at your hair colour. Is it golden blonde or light warm brown?

✓ Does your skin have golden undertones and maybe a few freckles as well?

✓ Are your eyes soft brown or soft hazel/moss?

✓ Do the colour test with orchid and peach, and then with sea green and olive: *go to page 33*. You should find that your best shade of pink is peach, while olive tones will suit you better than cooler blue-based sea greens.

Your secondary characteristic is warm. You will notice that all your additional colours have a warmth to them.

Your additional colours

As a Soft and Warm you can now add these 12 extra shades to your master palette. Mix darker colours with a similar colour but one or two tones lighter – for example, wear light charcoal with moss, chocolate with golden brown, or light navy with salmon.

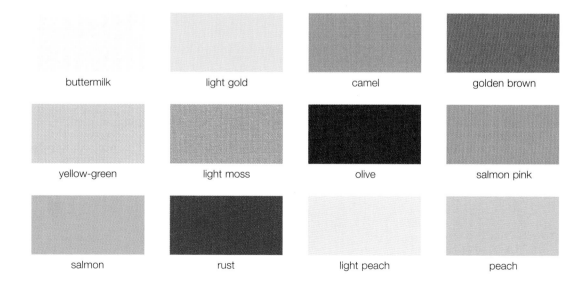

buttermilk	light gold	camel	golden brown
yellow-green	light moss	olive	salmon pink
salmon	rust	light peach	peach

Your face

✓ Your soft colouring needs to be complemented with make-up in soft, muted tones.

✓ For eye pencils try moss, brown or coffee.

✓ Accent eye shadows such as khaki, greyed green or brown will blend perfectly with peach, fawn or toffee.

✓ Your blusher will need to be soft and warm: try sienna.

✓ Soft lip pencils are best for you: use spice or natural.

✓ You will always need to wear lipstick to give you some definition. Balance your look with lipstick colours such as sandalwood, spiced peach or nutmeg. Try lip gloss as an alternative: a natural warm shade is good for you.

In your make-up bag

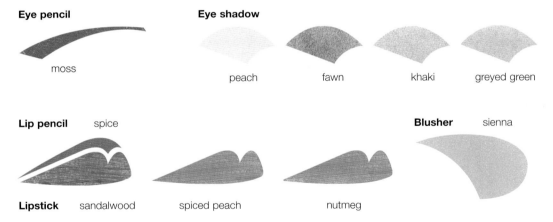

Eye pencil

moss

Eye shadow

peach   fawn   khaki   greyed green

Lip pencil   spice

Blusher   sienna

Lipstick   sandalwood   spiced peach   nutmeg

Your hair

✓ Your hair will be dark blonde or light to medium brown. If you highlight your hair, keep the colours warm and golden. A mix of hair colours will also work well for you: add rich warm gold or copper tones to enhance the richness of the colour.

✓ When natural grey highlights appear, just carry on adding the highlights or lowlights as you have been doing. You can go golden, but if you change your hair colour completely, your dominant colouring will change, too.

Mixing colours with confidence
Soft & warm

Warm weather combinations

business wear

sage + salmon

camel + natural beige

cocoa + peach

verbena + light moss

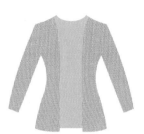

casual wear

rust + shell

jade + light moss

taupe + golden brown

yellow-green + greyed green

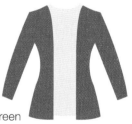

special occasion wear

peach + salmon

salmon pink + rust

light moss + olive

light gold + buttermilk

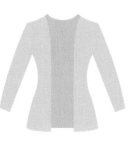

Cool weather combinations

business wear

chocolate + golden brown

teal + camel

olive + light moss

charcoal + salmon pink

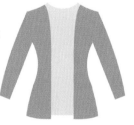

casual wear

turquoise + yellow-green

spruce + rust

pewter + camel

cocoa + light gold

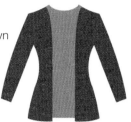

special occasion wear

claret + salmon pink

jade + teal

damson + olive

rose beige + peach

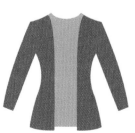

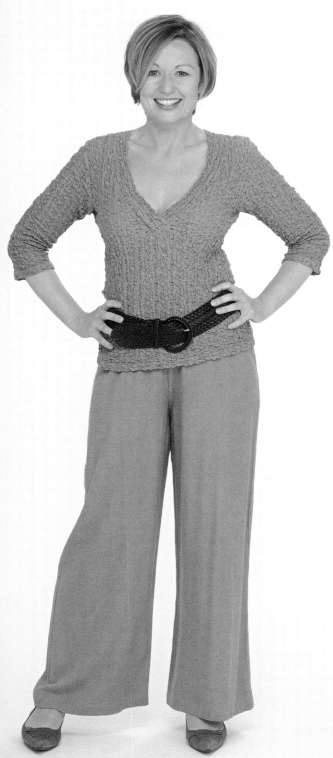

Rose brown worn tone on tone is perfect for someone who is Soft and Warm.

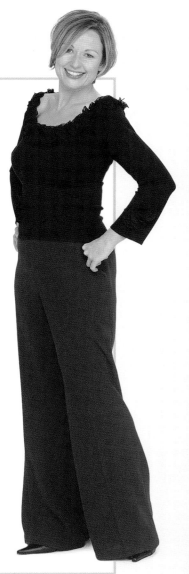

How to wear black

Black is quite a deep shade for you as lighter colours suit you better. Always wear black away from your face and choose fabrics that are textured or soft to the touch, such as knits. Details such as frills, velvet or chiffon trims, ribbons and bows will all help to soften the look. Keep your make-up colours soft and warm and do not be tempted to go too dark with your eye shadow. A little shimmer on the eyelids will give your face a natural lift. Gold jewellery and coloured beads will soften the overall effect.

Now that you know your colour palette, find out how to reflect your style through colour: *go to pages 138–155.*

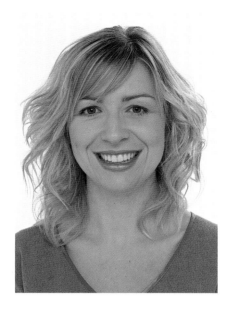

Soft & cool

✓ Take a close look at your hair colour. Would you describe it as ash blonde or cool brown?

✓ Does your skin have a slightly pink tone? Do you tend to blush easily?

✓ Do you have smoky blue, green or grey eyes?

✓ Do the colour test with peach and orchid, and then with olive and sea green: *go to page 33*. You should find that your best pink is a cool shade such as orchid, and the cool tones of sea green will suit you better than warmer olive.

Your secondary characteristic is cool. Your additional colours will add coolness and depth to your main colour palette.

Your additional colours

As a Soft and Cool you can now add these 12 extra shades to your master palette. When your are wearing warm colours like chocolate, rose brown or verbena, mix them with cooler shades such as lavender, soft fuchsia or eau de nil.

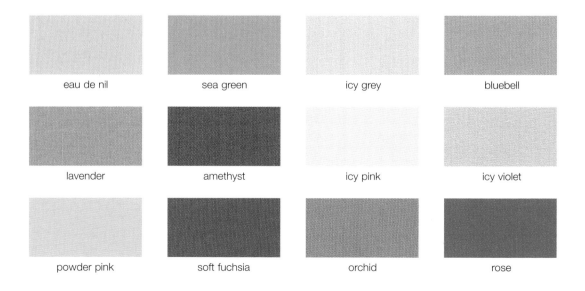

eau de nil	sea green	icy grey	bluebell
lavender	amethyst	icy pink	icy violet
powder pink	soft fuchsia	orchid	rose

Your face

✓ Your soft colouring needs to be complemented with cool, muted make-up shades; avoid using colour combinations that are too contrasting.

✓ For eye pencils try coffee, aubergine, granite or dark blue.

✓ Accent eye shadows such as cocoa, delph, heather or smoky blues and greys work well with melon, dusk, pale pinks and greys.

✓ Your blusher will need to be soft and cool: try rose or candy pink.

✓ Cool shades of lip pencil work best, so try natural or pink.

✓ Balance your whole look with soft cool lipsticks like mulberry, soft mauve or dusty rose. Lip gloss also works well for you: try pink shell.

In your make-up bag

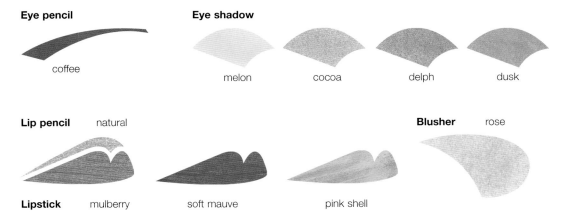

Eye pencil

coffee

Eye shadow

melon   cocoa   delph   dusk

Lip pencil   natural

Lipstick   mulberry   soft mauve   pink shell

Blusher   rose

Your hair

✓ You will have dark blonde to light or medium brown hair that has ash, rather than honey-coloured, undertones to it.

✓ You will probably already be highlighting your hair; keep to cool platinum or ash shades and avoid red or coppery tones.

✓ When natural grey highlights appear, just carry on adding the highlights or lowlights as you have been doing.

Mixing colours with confidence
Soft & cool

Warm weather combinations

business wear

charcoal blue + bluebell

jade + sea green

taupe + icy grey

light periwinkle + lavender

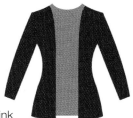

casual wear

sky blue + eau de nil

blush pink + rose

shell + rose brown

emerald turquoise + turquoise

special occasion wear

rose + powder pink

light periwinkle + icy grey

sage + greyed green

soft violet + icy violet

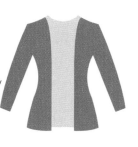

Cool weather combinations

business wear

light navy + orchid

charcoal + amethyst

teal + jade

rose brown + powder pink

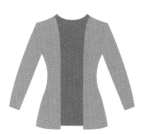

casual wear

blush pink + rose

damson + amethyst

spruce + sage

charcoal + soft fuchsia

special occasion wear

amethyst + lavender

sapphire + bluebell

claret + orchid

emerald turquoise + sea green

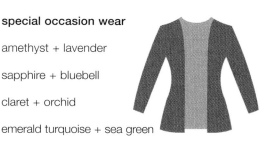

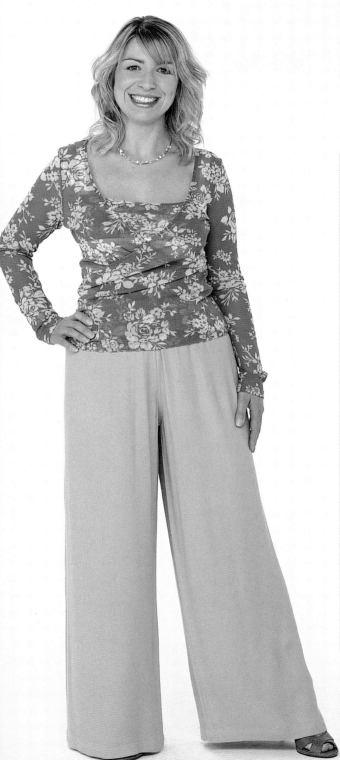

A perfect combination for someone who is Soft and Cool is soft powder pink and cocoa.

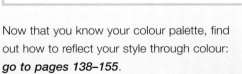

How to wear black

Black is not in your palette, but a textured fabric will soften the colour. For example, a black and white tweed will have the overall appearance of grey. You can also soften a plain black jacket by wearing it with a top in amethyst, lavender or icy grey. When wearing a black top, choose a V or round neck to ensure that the colour is not close to your face. Keep make-up colours soft and cool – a soft pink lipstick, a soft-coloured eye pencil, like granite, and a subtle rose blush. Silver and pearls work well with black for evening.

Now that you know your colour palette, find out how to reflect your style through colour: *go to pages 138–155*.

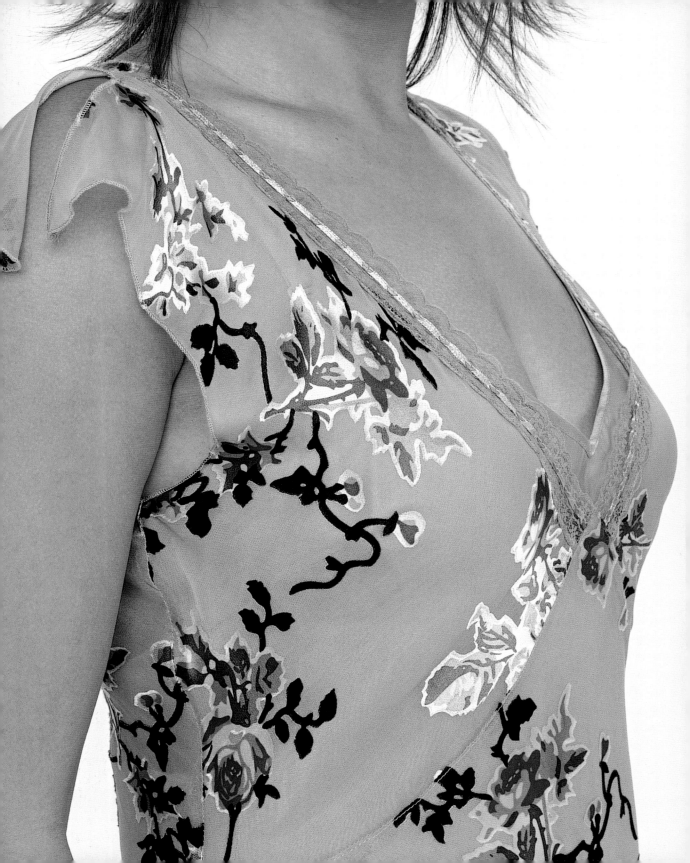

3

size doesn't matter, shape does

Women should have curves

While fashion magazines may be full of waif-like models with fragile, stick-thin limbs and bodies as flat as boards, women are actually designed to have curves. It's natural, it's feminine, it's sexy – and most men say they prefer curvy women.

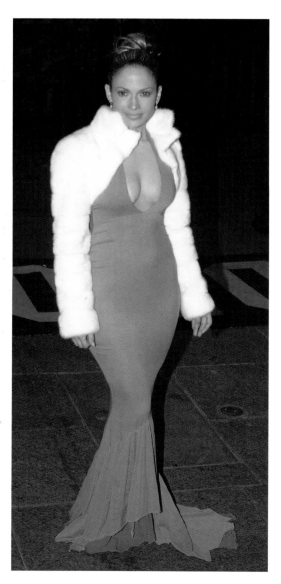

When it comes to looking good, it's not your size or shape that matters, it's the fit of your clothes. Wearing the right clothes is not about following the latest fashion or fad, it's about choosing what actually suits you – not your best friend – and what makes you feel comfortable and confident.

By knowing your basic body shape and understanding the guidelines for choosing the types of clothes that will accentuate your good features and minimize your less-than-perfect areas, you will be able to dress in the way that suits you best. You will also be able to see how to make subtle changes to the way you put your wardrobe together.

Today, the choice of clothes is so varied that you should always be able to find something that will complement your body shape, scale, proportions and colouring.

Body shapes

Clothing is either constructed along straight lines, which give a garment a more rigid, structured form, or along curved lines, which give a more fluid shape that tends to follow the curves of the body.

You cannot alter your basic body line by diet or exercise. It will remain essentially the

Jennifer Lopez is widely admired for her fantastic hourglass curves and shapely derrière.

same throughout your life because your body line is based on your skeleton as well as your genes. The distribution of body fat is also dependent on your genes. If you have a tendency to carry extra weight on your hips, you will almost certainly have a proportionally smaller waist; conversely, women who carry extra weight around their tummies will have straight hips and bottoms.

Biologically, women are designed to carry more fat beneath their skin than men (the original hunter-gatherers), and we actually need a few curves in order for our bodies to work efficiently. Fatty deposits around the hips, legs and arms should not be viewed as worrying health indicators (unless you are grossly overweight).

When most women stand in front of a mirror, they focus on all the things they would like to change about their bodies. On the following pages, you will learn how to recognize your assets and show them off, and how to play down the parts of your body that you are not so happy with. The objective is for you to understand your shape, to be positive about it and to make the most of what nature has given you.

Whether you are petite or have a fuller figure, the cut of the clothes that will flatter you the best will depend on your basic body shape. For example, if you have a Full Hourglass figure, wearing softer lines is recommended. The only difference between what suits a petite or fuller-figured woman of this body shape will be the size of the pattern and the weight of the fabric in which the garment is made.

The illusion of a balanced body

When choosing clothes, your aim is to create the illusion of having a balanced body: a Neat Hourglass figure with:

✓ **Shoulders and hips in line**

✓ **A defined bust**

✓ **A waist, even with a softly curved tummy**

✓ **A curved bottom**

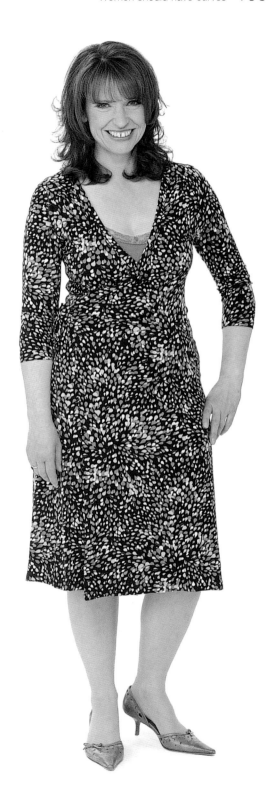

What body shape are you?

To identify your basic body shape, answer the questions in the boxes below. If you don't fit exactly into just one shape, choose the one that most closely resembles you. Then turn to the relevant section to discover your clothing guidelines.

Neat Hourglass

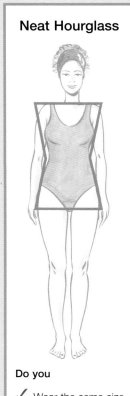

Do you

- ✓ Wear the same size top and bottom?
- ✓ Have a clearly defined waist?
- ✓ Have a clearly defined bust?
- ✓ Have a curved bottom?

go to pages 112–113

Full Hourglass

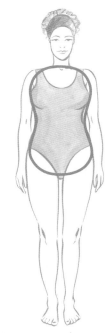

Do you

- ✓ Buy a slightly larger top for your bust?
- ✓ Find that waistbands are often too large?
- ✓ Find that a straight skirt rises up?
- ✓ Feel most comfortable in more fluid fabrics?

go to pages 114–115

Triangle

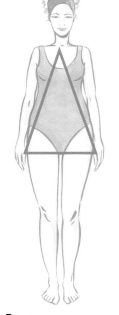

Do you

- ✓ Wear a larger size on your bottom half than your top?
- ✓ Have a clearly defined waist?
- ✓ Have narrower shoulders than hips?
- ✓ Carry weight on your hips or thighs?

go to pages 116–117

Inverted Triangle

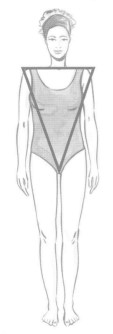

Do you

✓ Wear a larger size on your top half than your bottom?

✓ Have wider shoulders than hips?

✓ Have a straight ribcage?

✓ Prefer an uncluttered look?

go to pages 118–119

Lean Column

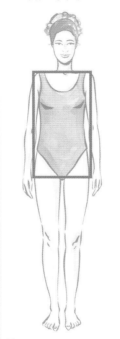

Do you

✓ Wear the same size on your top and bottom halves?

✓ Have a minimal bust?

✓ Have little waist definition?

✓ Have flat hips and bottom?

go to pages 120–121

Rectangle

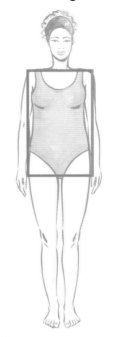

Do you

✓ Have shoulders and hips in line?

✓ Have no waist definition?

✓ Have flat hips and bottom?

✓ Carry any extra weight around your middle?

go to pages 122–123

Round

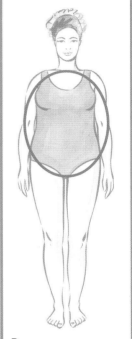

Do you

✓ Have rounded shoulders?

✓ Have fullness in the tummy area?

✓ Have wonderful shapely legs?

✓ Feel uncomfortable when clothes are tucked in?

go to pages 124–125

Neat hourglass

Lucky you! You have a balanced body with your top half in proportion to your bottom half. This means that your clothes don't need to work hard at evening out your shape and can simply follow your natural curves.

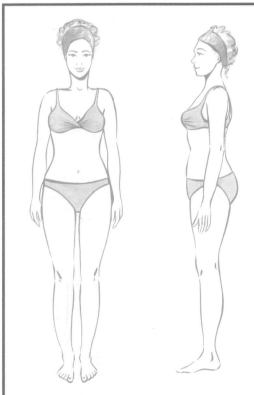

Your build is characterized by:

✓ A defined bust

✓ A defined waist

✓ A neat bottom

✓ Neat hips

Your golden rules

✓ Show off your body by wearing clothes that define your waist, enhance your bust and highlight your hips and bottom.

✗ Avoid wearing clothes that hide your body line, or you risk looking an extra three to four kilos (six to ten pounds) heavier than you are.

Your clothing lines

Jackets	Fitted, with waist definition.
Tops	Shaped, crossovers or wraps.
Skirts	Straight, panelled, flip, bias cut, soft pleats or full, preferably with a waistband and some shaping (darts) over the hips and bottom.
Trousers	Any type, with a waistband (see above).
Jeans	Designed for women's bodies.
Dresses	Any style, either shaped or belted.
Coats	All shapes, as long as they have some shape at the waist or a belt.
Swimwear	As long as your proportions are good, you can wear any style (see illustration left).

Your best fabrics

Choose fabrics that are light to medium in weight
and texture. These will skim the curves of your body:

Cotton
Linen
Silk
Tightly woven gabardine to relaxed wool crepe
All jerseys and polyesters
All knits

Your best patterns

Because the top and bottom half of your body are in
balance, you are able to wear most types of pattern.

Stripes
Abstract
Checks
Spots
Florals
Paisleys

You should avoid

Boxy jackets
Trousers or skirts that have no shaping
Straight tunics
Men's shirts
Baggy sweaters and sportswear
Too much layering

For more on proportion and scale:
go to pages 130–132; for more on who
can wear what: *go to pages 126–129*.

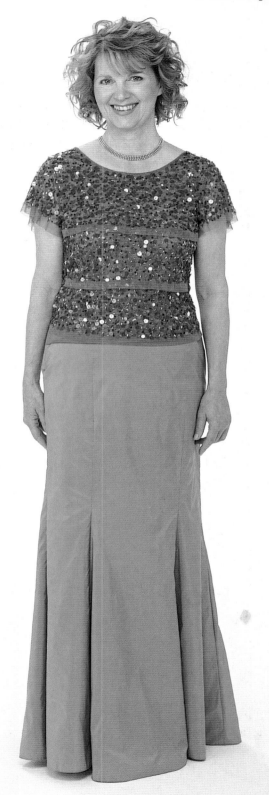

Full hourglass

Lucky you! You have the most feminine body shape with full curves in all the right places. By choosing clothes that are fluid and shaped, you will be able to accentuate your curves rather than cover them up.

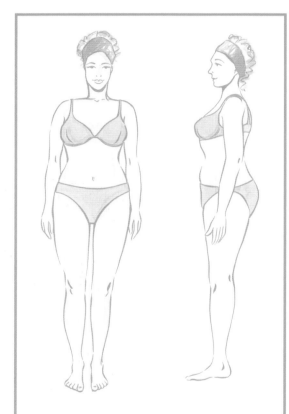

Your build is characterized by:

✓ A full bust

✓ A small waist

✓ A rounded bottom

✓ Rounded hips

Your golden rules

✓ It is important that you wear clothes that follow your body line as opposed to those that constrict you.

✓ Choose fabrics carefully. Avoid heavy or stiff materials or you'll end up with tops and jackets that are two to three sizes bigger than you need just to accommodate your curves.

Your clothing lines

Jackets	Shaped, with shawl collars or concealed front openings.
Tops	Shaped, crossovers or wraps, in soft fabrics.
Skirts	Flip, bias or full, and adjustable at the waist
Trousers	Flat-fronted with side zip.
Dresses	Shaped, wrap or bias-cut shift.
Coats	Shawl collar, single-breasted or shaped.
Swimwear	Underwiring or support is essential. Avoid stripes and detailing at the bust and hips (see illustration left).

Your best fabrics

Should be light to medium weight, with little texture.
If choosing cotton or linen, look for fabrics cut on the
bias to give movement and accommodate your curves:

Silk and chiffon
Relaxed wool crepe
All jerseys and polyesters
Fine knits
Fabric that gives and stretches
Lycra, the best friend of the Full Hourglass

Your best patterns

Avoid geometric patterns, as lines will not lie straight over
your curves. Instead, opt for more fluid shapes such as:

Spots
Florals
Paisleys
Circles and squiggles

You should avoid

Jeans (too many pockets)
Straight skirts, except in soft fabrics with some Lycra
Boxy, double-breasted jackets
Straight tunics
Front-opening shirts and blouses
Baggy sweaters and sportswear
Too much layering
Crisp fabrics
Stripes and checks

For more on proportion and scale:
go to pages 130–132; for more on who
can wear what: *go to pages 126–129.*

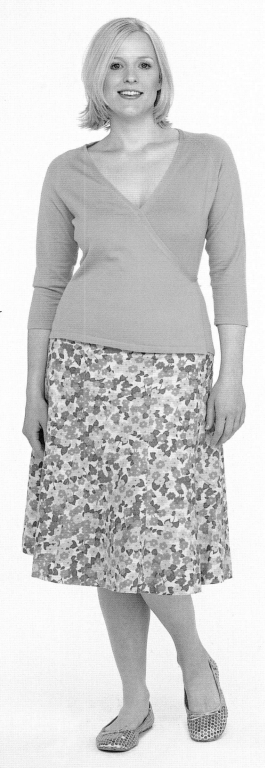

Triangle

Lucky you! You can bring all the attention to the top half of your body. You are often referred to as pear-shaped, so with your choice of clothes you should aim to accentuate your bust and minimize your bottom and hips.

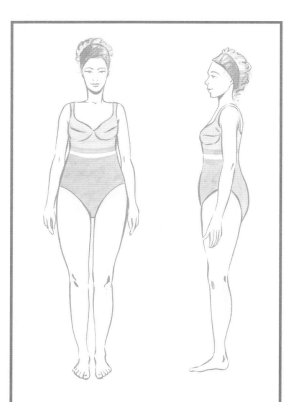

Your golden rules

✓ Your jackets and tops need to finish either above or below the widest point of your hips and bottom.

✓ Layering on your top half creates visual interest and draws the eye upwards.

✓ Buy jackets or tops that fit your shoulders rather than your hips – you can always leave the bottom button undone.

Your clothing lines

Jackets	Details, collars, pockets, buttons or double-breasted are excellent.
Tops	Patterned, horizontal stripes or twin-sets.
Skirts	Simple lines: long flip, bias cut or panelled.
Trousers	Plain, flat-fronted with side zip, bootleg or flared (for long legs).
Dresses	Separates work better.
Coats	Square shoulders or wide collars.
Swimwear	Keep detailing above the waist. Beware of high-cut styles that finish at your widest point (see illustration left).

Your build is characterized by:

✓ Full hips or thighs

✓ A defined waist

✓ Shoulders that may slope and are narrower than your hips

✓ A top half that appears small

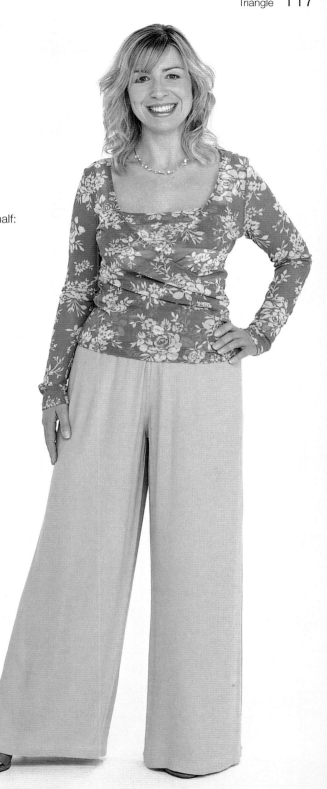

Your best fabrics

Your aim is to balance out your body shape, so certain fabrics will work best on your lower half:

Light- to medium-weight fabrics with minimum texture
Soft, fluid fabrics that drape easily, such as wool crepe, jersey, knits, fabrics cut on the bias, silks

Other fabrics will flatter and draw attention to your top half:

Light fabrics worn layered
Medium- to heavyweight fabrics
Texture, which adds volume
Cotton and linen
All types of woollen fabrics
Crisper fabrics, which add bulk

Your best patterns

Any pattern, such as florals and horizontal stripes, is a great way to draw attention to the upper half of your body. Always wear plain colours below the waist.

You should avoid

Jeans (too many pockets)
Straight skirts
Details on skirts and trousers
Halternecks and raglan sleeves
Tight-fitting single-layered tops
Tops and jackets that finish at your widest point

For more on proportion and scale:
go to pages 130–132; for more on who can wear what: *go to pages 126–129*.

Inverted triangle

Lucky you! You have great shoulders – halternecks are made for you.
To balance the upper and lower parts of your body, you need to highlight
your hips and bottom, focussing all attention below your waist.

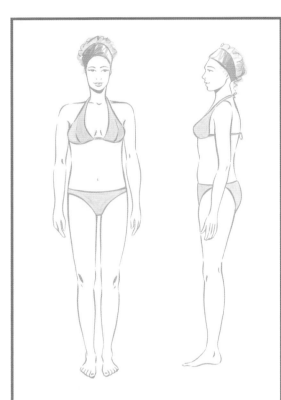

Your build is characterized by:

✓ Straight and squared shoulder line

✓ Little definition between waist/hips

✓ Flat hips and bottom

✓ A bottom half that seems smaller
than your top half

Your golden rules

✓ You will need to ensure that there is
minimum detail on your shoulder line;
keep this area as simple as possible.

✓ Your clothing line needs to be straight
and clean.

✓ Your silhouette should be uncluttered.

Your clothing lines

Jackets   Constructed, or shaped with
angular lines (revered collars).

Tops   Simple lines.

Skirts   Straight, box pleats or panelled.

Trousers   Any style – pockets and details
will accentuate your bottom.

Dresses   Simple straight lines, or shifts.

Coats   Straight lines with a slightly
shaped waistline.

Swimwear   Halter and square necklines
work well, as do details on the
hips (see illustration left). Avoid
floral patterns. Go for styles
where tops and bottoms are
sold separately.

Your best fabrics

Crisp, constructed fabrics work best for you because your body line is straight and angled.

Crisp cottons and linens
Gabardine and fine wool
Satins and crisp silks
Crinkled fabrics

Your best patterns

You can wear patterns above and below the waistline but they must be geometric to balance the clothing line.

Stripes
Checks
Geometrics
Squiggles and spots

You should avoid

Frills and flounces
Gathered waistlines
Tiered skirts
Epaulettes
Soft, floppy and fluffy fabrics
Bias cuts

For more on proportion and scale: *go to pages 130–132*; for more on who can wear what: *go to pages 126–129*.

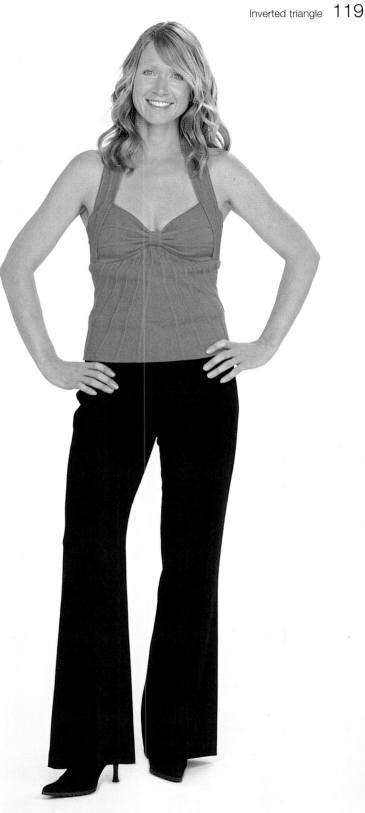

Lean column

Lucky you! You've got the figure of a catwalk model. Your challenge is to create an illusion of curves where there are none, so go for designs with shape and detail that emphasize your bust, hips and bottom and define your waist.

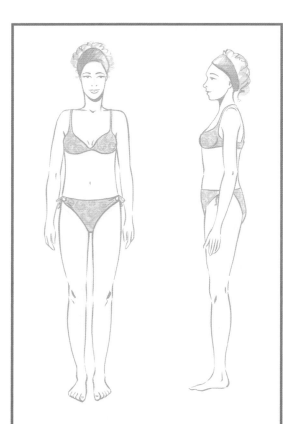

Your build is characterized by:

✓ Narrow shoulders and lean limbs

✓ Flat chest or small bust

✓ Small and non-defined waist

✓ Narrow hips and flat bottom

Your golden rules

✓ Highlight your hips and bottom.

✓ Enhance your bust line with details.

✓ Your clothing line needs to be straight, with emphasis on the waist.

✓ Use texture and layering.

Your clothing lines

Jackets	Waisted jackets, with details or pockets.
Tops	Details, textures, patterns and layers.
Skirts	A-line, panelled, gored or pleated.
Trousers	Shaped, pleated and pocketed.
Dresses	Princess line with curved darts and details.
Coats	Martingale, shaped.
Swimwear	Padded styles are perfect. Use patterned two-pieces to emphasize your bust and hips (see illustration left). Vertical chevron lines on a one-piece will give the illusion of shape.

Your best fabrics

Textured fabrics or fabrics that you can layer
are both good choices for you.

Cottons and linens
Gabardine, fine wool and lightweight tweeds
Satins and silks
Crinkled fabrics
Light woven textures

Your best patterns

Wearing pattern on your top half will draw the
eye and emphasize your bust, while clothing
details such as pockets will accentuate your hips.

Squiggles, paisleys and spots
Horizontal stripes
Checks
Geometrics
Discreet florals

You should avoid

Full frills and flounces
Large, gathered skirts
Belted jackets and coats
Bulky, heavy textures
Close fitting, figure-hugging garments

For more on proportion and scale:
go to pages 130–132; for more on who
can wear what: *go to pages 126–129*.

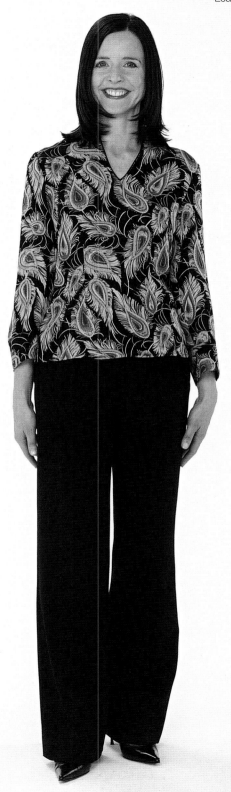

Rectangle

Lucky you! You are the one with flat hips and a flat bottom. However, some Rectangles will have a fuller bust, giving a softer edge to their shape. Your main aim is to soften those edges even more and create the appearance of curves.

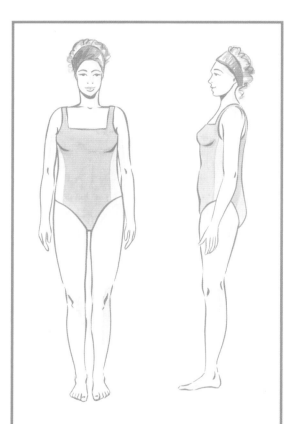

Your build is characterized by:

✓ Straight shoulder line

✓ Straight hips and bottom

✓ Very little waist definition

✓ Straight ribcage

Your golden rules

✓ Use details on your hips and bottom to create shape.

✓ Avoid details at the waist, such as noticeable waistbands or belts.

✓ Keep your clothing line straight.

✓ Go for the uncluttered look.

Your clothing lines

Jackets   Structured and shaped.

Tops   Simple, clean lines.

Skirts   Crossover, straight, box pleats or panelled.

Trousers   The choice is yours.

Dresses   Simple straight lines or shifts.

Coats   Straight lines with some emphasis on the waist.

Swimwear   On a one-piece, a central panel in a darker shade gives the illusion of a slimmer shape, as do square necklines (see illustration left). Avoid high-waisted bikini bottoms and choose geometric patterns.

Your best fabrics

Most Rectangles can wear crisp fabrics, but if you have a full bust, slightly softer fabrics work better.

Wool crepe and woven wool
Cottons and linens
Jersey and lightweight tweeds
Fine knits

Your best patterns

Geometric patterns work best for you because your body is straight.

Vertical stripes
Checks
Geometrics
Squiggles and spots

You should avoid

Frills and flounces
Gathered waistlines
Soft, floppy and fluffy fabrics
Bias cuts
Belted jackets and coats
Florals and paisleys

For more on proportion and scale: *go to pages 130–132*; for more on who can wear what: *go to pages 126–129*.

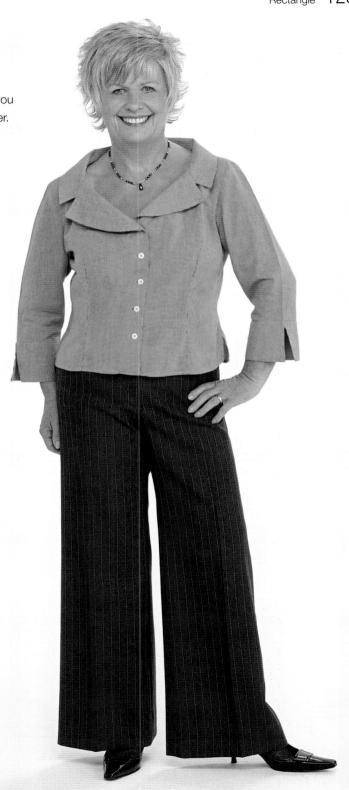

Round

Lucky you! You've got great legs. Your problem area is your central torso, so wherever possible use accessories to draw the eye to the area above your bust and below your hips. Your aim is to give the impression of a slightly longer body.

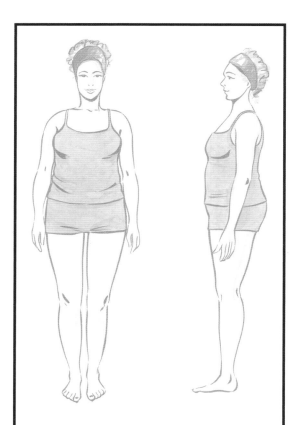

Your build is characterized by:

✓ Rounded shoulder line

✓ Curved back

✓ Fullness around the middle

✓ Flattish bottom

Your golden rules

✓ Make sure your clothes hang from your shoulders.

✓ Clothing lines need to be straight, and fabrics soft to avoid any unnecessary volume or bulkiness.

✓ Keep any detail above the bust line and below the hip line.

✓ Accessorize, accessorize, accessorize.

Your clothing lines

Jackets	Cardigan-style, collarless, shawl collar, V-shaped neckline.
Tops	Simple lines, no details.
Skirts	Wrap, flip or panelled.
Trousers	Drawstrings, no waistband.
Dresses	A-line (trapeze).
Coats	A-line, cardigan-style.
Swimwear	Try a tankini or vest top that covers the middle and isn't too figure-hugging (see illustration left). For more cover use a sarong. Details on the shoulders draw the eye towards your face.

Your best fabrics

The key is to choose soft, fluid fabrics that hang well and don't cling or hug the figure. Stiff or thick fabric will add unwelcome girth.

Soft cottons and linens
Wool crepe
Jersey
Knits
Silks

Your best patterns

Try to go for muted and subtle patterns as much as possible; anything too bold will overpower.

Soft or faded stripes
Squiggles and spots
Abstract florals or paisleys

You should avoid

Stiff fabrics
Pockets
Gathered waistlines or any other details
   over the tummy area
Sharp angular details such as lapels
Vibrant and dramatic patterns over the torso

For more on proportion and scale: *go to pages 130–132*; for more on who can wear what: *go to pages 126–129*.

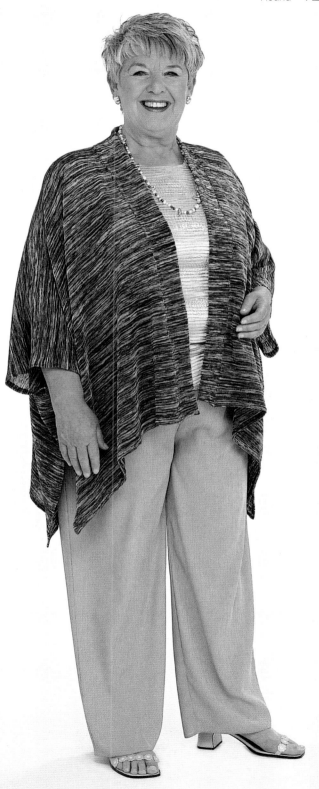

Who can wear what

By appreciating the subtle differences in the styling of clothes, you will be able to choose exactly the right type of jacket, skirt, top and so on to flatter your body shape and so enhance your overall look.

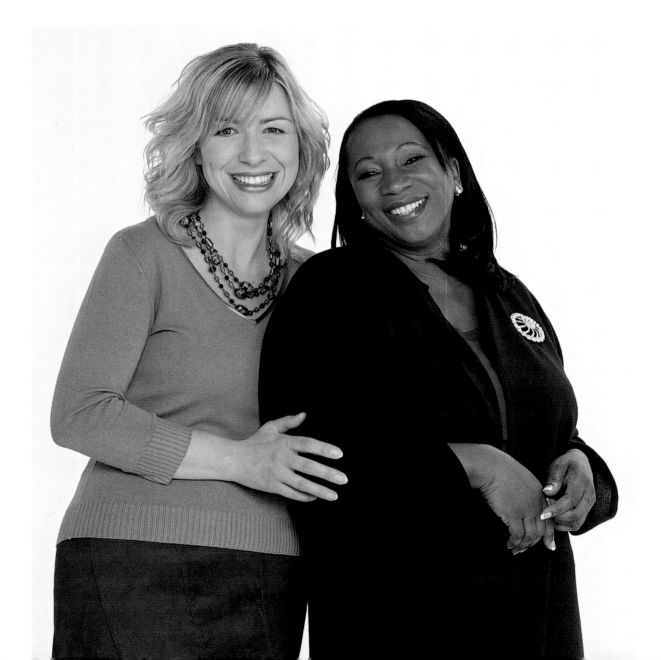

Jackets

1 Shaped Suit most body shapes. Good for emphasizing or enhancing waistlines.

2 Shawl collar Best on soft and rounded body lines such as Full Hourglasses and Rounds. Make sure there are no buttons at a wide point such as the bust line.

3 Fitted Great for Neat Hourglass and Lean Column shapes, as long as they're not too tight. Good for Inverted Triangles if they have angled revers and straight seams.

4 Boxy, no pockets Good for Inverted Triangles, Lean Columns and Rectangles.

5 Double-breasted Great for Triangles, but not long blazer styles.

6 Straight cardigan Best look for Rounds, especially in soft fabrics.

Tops

1 Wrap Good for Neat and Full Hourglass shapes.

2 Patterned Suit Triangles and Lean Columns who need detail on their top half.

3 Simple line A must for everyone.

4 Detailed top For women with small busts, Triangles and Lean Columns. Avoid if full busted.

5 Twin set For all body shapes.

6 Shirt Great for all medium- to small-busted body shapes, except Full Hourglass and Round.

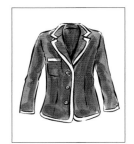

1

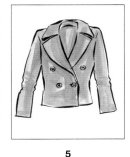

2

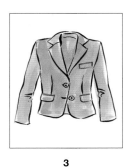

3

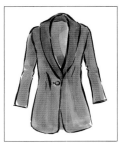

4

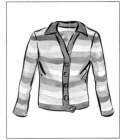

5

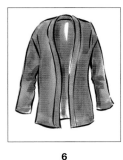

6

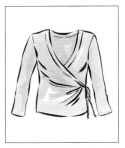

1

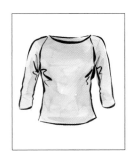

2

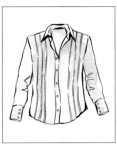

3

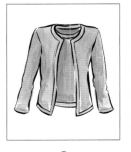

4

5

6

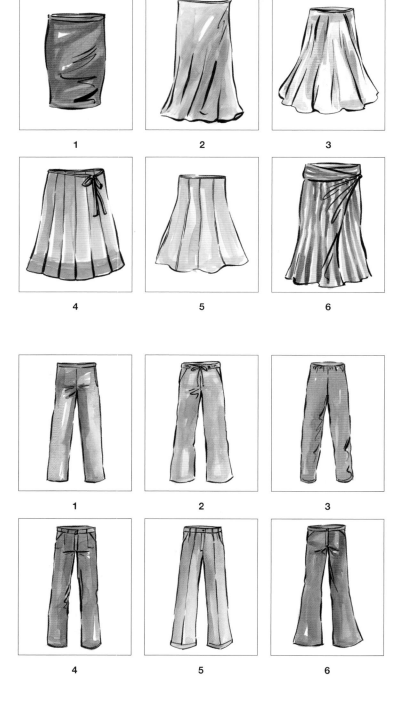

Skirts

1 Straight, short Good for Rectangles, Inverted Triangles and Neat Hourglasses.

2 Bias cut For Neat and Full Hourglasses and Triangles. Make sure the side seams hang straight.

3 Full Long legs are needed, but best for Neat and Full Hourglasses.

4 Box pleats Great for Rectangles and Inverted Triangles with flat hips.

5 Panelled Works on all shapes. If you have curvy hips, use soft fabrics.

6 Wrap/Crossover Good for any shape where the waistline might need adjusting.

Trousers

1 Plain fronted, side zip Suit every body shape.

2 Drawstring Great for fluctuating waists. Work well on Triangles with small waists, Rectangles with no waists, and Full Hourglasses.

3 No waistband Best for Rounds and Rectangles, and high waists.

4 Jeans Best worn by Inverted Triangles, Lean Columns and Rectangles with small bottoms.

5 High waisted with pleats Good for Lean Columns and those who are long-bodied with narrow hips.

6 Flares Long legs needed, or with high-heeled shoes or boots.

Dresses

1 Shift Best on Lean Columns, Rectangles and Inverted Triangles.

2 Wrap A winner on Neat and Full Hourglass shapes and pregnant women.

3 Bias cut Curves are essential for this shape, so good for Full and Neat Hourglasses and Triangles with curvy hips.

4 Empire line Great for long-waisted bodies.

5 Belted A waist in the right place is essential, so avoid if you are high or low waisted.

6 A-line A great look for Rounds but avoid if you are a Triangle.

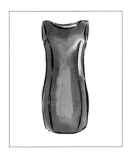

1

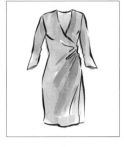

2

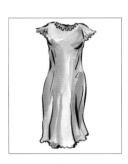

3

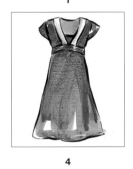

4

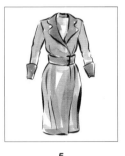

5

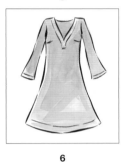

6

Coats

1 Belted You need to be tall and have a well-defined waist to wear this style of coat. Particularly good for Neat Hourglasses.

2 Swing A great look for Rounds.

3 Singled-breasted, no pockets This style will suit everyone.

4 Double-breasted, collar For Triangles, and Lean Columns and Rectangles provided you are not full busted.

5 Single-breasted shawl collar Best on Neat and Full Hourglasses.

6 Cardigan style Looks particularly good on Full Hourglass and Round shapes.

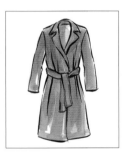

1

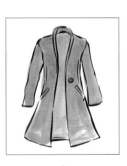

2

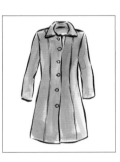

3

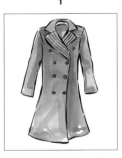

4

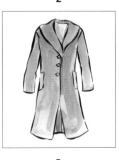

5

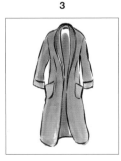

6

Proportions

When you look at proportions, you are considering the relationship of your body to your legs, as well as the position of your waist. Once you understand your body proportions, you'll be able to combine clothes that appear to adjust any imbalances and give the illusion of perfect proportions.

The possible combinations

High waisted + short rise + long legs
High waisted + long rise + average to short legs
Low waisted + short rise + average to short legs
Low waisted + long rise + short legs
Balanced waist + balanced rise + balanced legs

Finding out your proportions

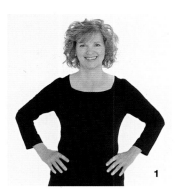
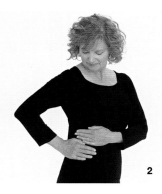

Balanced waist

Balanced rise + legs
You are extremely lucky in having perfect proportions, with the length of your body and legs in balance with each other. Remember what your height, scale and body shape are and follow the guidelines given in the appropriate section of this book (pages 110–129) whenever you go clothes shopping. This will ensure that you only buy what suits you the best.

Stand in front of a mirror so that you can see your silhouette. Place your hands on your natural waistline **(1)**. Then place the flat of one hand underneath your bust, and the other below the first hand **(2)**. If you can easily place two hands widthways between your bust and waistline, you are low-waisted and may be slightly shorter on the leg. If you have a struggle to get the second hand in, you have long legs and may be high-waisted. If you can get approximately 1½ hands in, you have perfect proportions.

You may be high-waisted but feel that your legs are not particularly long. If so, view yourself from the back; it's possible that you are long in the 'rise' (the measurement between waistline and crotch). Conversely, you could be short in this area.

High waisted

Short rise + long legs

Create the illusion of lowering your waist:

✓ Dropped waistlines or hipsters.

✓ Skirts and trousers without waistbands.

✓ Low-slung belts.

✓ Long jackets and tops.

✓ Volume or pattern on your legs.

✓ Long tops and long skirts.

✗ Don't tuck in tops.

Long rise + average to short legs

Create the illusion of lowering your waist without shortening your legs:

✓ Low waistlines or hipsters.

✓ Skirts and trousers without waistbands.

✓ Low-slung belts.

✓ High heels

✓ Long jackets and tops with narrow skirts or trousers.

✗ Don't clutter your leg area.

✗ Don't tuck in tops.

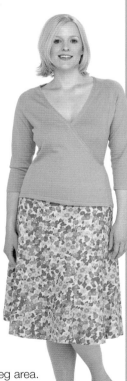

Low waisted

Short rise + average to short legs

Create the illusion of raising your waist without shortening your legs:

✓ Belts and tuck-ins.

✓ Short tops.

✓ Minimal details in the rise area.

✓ Short jackets with long or short skirts.

✓ Straight-waisted or belted dresses.

✓ Long jackets with short skirts or narrow trousers.

✓ High heels.

✗ Don't clutter your leg area.

Long rise + short legs

Create the illusion of raising your waist and lengthening your legs:

✓ Belts and tuck-ins.

✓ Short tops and jackets.

✓ Details such as pockets or trims in the rise area.

✓ Keep to one colour from waist to toe.

✓ High heels.

✓ Straight-waisted or belted dresses.

✗ Don't clutter your leg area.

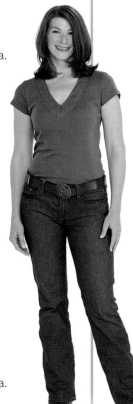

Scale

Scale is a combination of height and bone structure. Your scale may be petite, average or grand, and will determine the size of patterns, the weight of fabrics and how much texture you can wear, as well as the size of your accessories.

Petite

1.6m (5ft 3in) and under

✓ You're better wearing one colour from head to toe

✓ Two colours may be worn as long as the proportions are ⅔ to ⅓

✓ Best not to wear too much volume, as it will swamp you

Scale

You have:

✓ fine fingers, narrow wrists and ankles

✓ small facial features

✓ shoe size under 37

You should wear:

✓ smaller print patterns

✓ smaller accessories

✓ minimal texture and bulk

✓ neat hairstyles

Average

1.6–1.7m (5ft 3in–5ft 6in)

✓ You have the freedom to do what you like, as long as you follow your body shape (pages 110–125) and proportions (pages 130–131)

Scale

You have:

✓ neither petite nor grand bone structure

✓ shoe size between 37 and 40

You should wear:

✓ accessories that balance your scale (neither tiny nor extra-large)

✓ average-sized patterns

✓ either a 'wow' piece of clothing to make a statement or a single accessory such as a bag or a piece of jewellery

Grand

1.7m (5ft 6in) and over

✓ You need to use colour to break up your height

✓ By wearing differently proportioned clothes you will look more balanced (short jacket + short skirt will not do)

Scale

You have:

✓ large hands and feet, strong bone structure

✓ shoe size 40+

You should wear:

✓ larger, bolder prints

✓ statement accessories

✓ heavier weighted fabrics (or finer fabrics worn layered)

Flattering colour combinations

Now you know your best colours, you can combine them to create the look of a balanced body. Lighter or brighter colours will always draw attention to the areas where they're worn. Below are some of the most frequently used combinations.

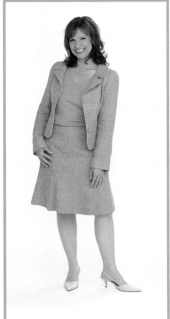

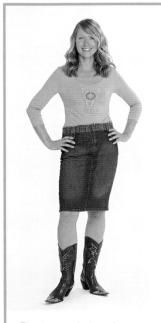

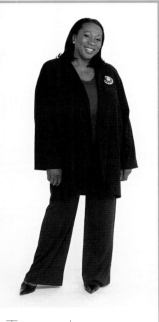

All-over colour

One colour used for the entire outfit or a single-coloured dress will give the appearance of height.

Colour blocks

Different blocks of colour on a jacket, top, skirt or trousers will give the appearance of reducing height.

Two colours

A jacket and skirt or trousers in one colour, with a top of another colour, is a great combination for everybody.

Other winning combinations

✓ A light top with a dark bottom will give the illusion of wider shoulders and slimmer hips, which is perfect for Triangles, but not for Inverted Triangles.

✓ A jacket in one colour, with a top and skirt or trousers in another, is a great combination for every body shape. If you are long in the body, you can break this look up with a belt.

✓ A dark top and light bottom will give the illusion of narrower shoulders and wider hips. This combination is excellent for Inverted Triangles but not for Triangles.

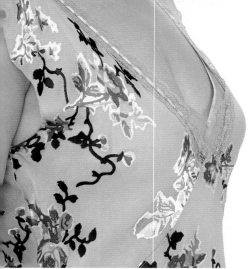

Clothing details

Your body shape and proportions will determine which clothing details, such as necklines, waistlines and sleeves, will flatter you the most. By learning to look at your body objectively, you will know how to buy clothes to suit your shape.

The golden rule

There is one golden rule that will ensure you are showing off your body shape to best advantage at all times: **never finish any part of a garment at the widest point of your body**. For example, you should avoid:

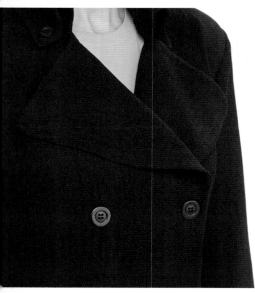

✗ jackets that finish at the widest point on your hips

✗ skirts that end at the fullest part of your legs

✗ short sleeves if you have a full bust

✗ short tops if you have a wide waist

Bust lines

If you don't wear the right bra, your clothes won't hang properly: **go to page 174** – the wrong bra can alter your body shape and clothing size. Have a variety of bras to suit different occasions and different tops.

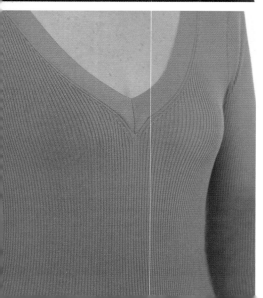

Small bust	Add details such as pockets, buttons, appliqué, ruffles or slogans. Texture and layering are also helpful. A padded bra always helps.
Full bust	Stick to simple cuts and plain fabrics (no heavy textures). A V-neck or jewel neckline is best for you. Front-opening shirts and blouses need to be worn with care, and should be made of soft or stretchy fabric.

Neck lines

When deciding which necklines to wear, be aware of how prominent your collarbones and/or your upper chest are, and of how confident you feel to reveal these parts of your body.

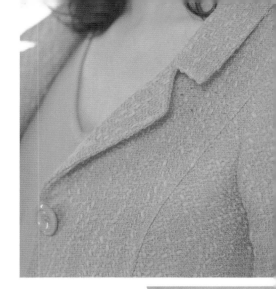

Boat/slash Give the illusion of wide shoulders. Good for Triangle shapes, but avoid if you have prominent collarbones or a scrawny neck.

Bardot Good for most shapes, but not if you have sloping shoulders.

V-necks Look good on everyone, and can always be accessorized. Plunging V-necks are elegant – but not if you have a long neck or if they reveal too much cleavage.

Scoop Work well on most women, particularly if you have narrow shoulders.

Cowl Perfect for full busts and softer body lines.

Roll Only if you have a long neck and no double chin.

Crew Suit most women, but they need to sit well.

Ruffles/frills Best for a longer neck and softer features.

Mandarin collars Not for those with a short neck or double chin.

Shirt collars Good for all women, and best worn open.

Jewel necklines Good for all.

Halternecks Excellent for Inverted Triangles.

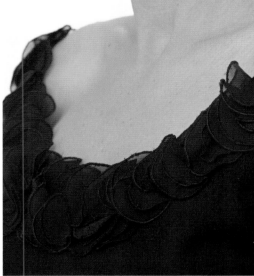

Shoulder lines

Inserted Good for all. If your shoulders slope or are rounded, consider shoulder pads.

Raglan You need a square shoulder line to wear these.

Dropped Good for adding width to the shoulders. They will also soften a strong shoulder line.

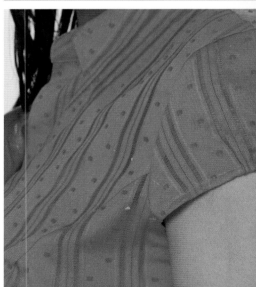

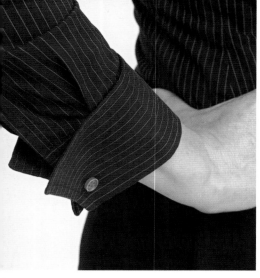

Sleeves

The key factor when choosing a sleeve length is to remember never to end the sleeves at a wide point on your arm.

Bracelet   Great for short to average arms.

Full   Best for average to long arms.

Batwing   Best worn by average to tall women.

Cuff details   Make sure that these do not overwhelm your hands.

Waist lines

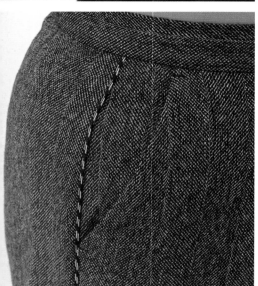

Create the illusion of a longer body by wearing a low waistline; to shorten your body, bring the waistline up.

Waistband   You need to have a clearly defined waist, as in Neat Hourglass, Full Hourglass and Triangle shapes, to wear trousers and skirts with waistbands. A wide waistband is excellent if you are long-waisted.

Elasticized   These may be your favourites if you have a fluctuating waistline. Best worn covered over but beware of adding bulk. Non-gathered elasticized waistbands are more flattering.

Dropped waist   Perfect for short-waisted women, but they don't work well for long-waisted women.

Hipsters   Good for short waists and those of you who do not have clearly defined waistlines (Inverted Triangles, Rectangles or Lean Columns).

Bottom lines

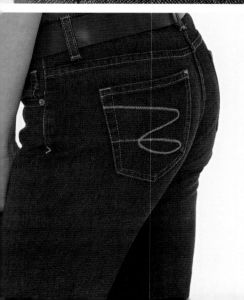

Decide where the widest part of your bottom is and avoid any details in that area. Instead of wearing a long jacket or top to hide your bottom, show off an asset such as your waist.

Tummy lines

Front pleats   Good if you have a flat tummy.

Zips   Front zips will add volume to your tummy; side and back zips will give a sleeker look.

Pockets   Pockets with flaps suit women with flat hips. Sloping pockets and pockets without flaps can be worn by everyone.

Belts   Great for averting the eye from a full waistline.

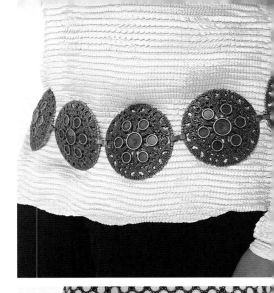

Thigh lines

If your thighs are wider than your hips, take care to avoid details in the thigh area. Looser fitting trousers and skirts are the answer.

Leg lines

Short legs   Wear skirts and trousers with minimal volume. Open-fronted shoes with a short skirt will add length to the leg, as will tights or socks in the same colour as your trousers or skirt. Avoid details and patterns.

Long legs   Wear skirts and trousers with lots of volume and detail. Patterns and layers are good for you.

Skinny legs   Add volume with textured tights and fabrics. Avoid anything too clingy.

Wide legs   Wear the same colour from waist to toes. Avoid anything too clingy or heavily textured. Loose and fluid fits work well.

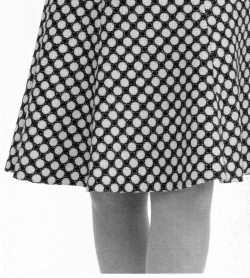

Ankle lines

Thin   Add details such as ankle straps, socks or different textures.

Wide   Go for open-fronted shoes.

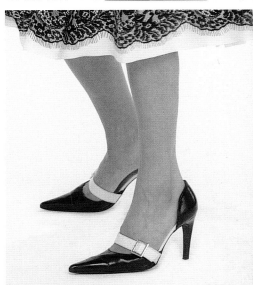

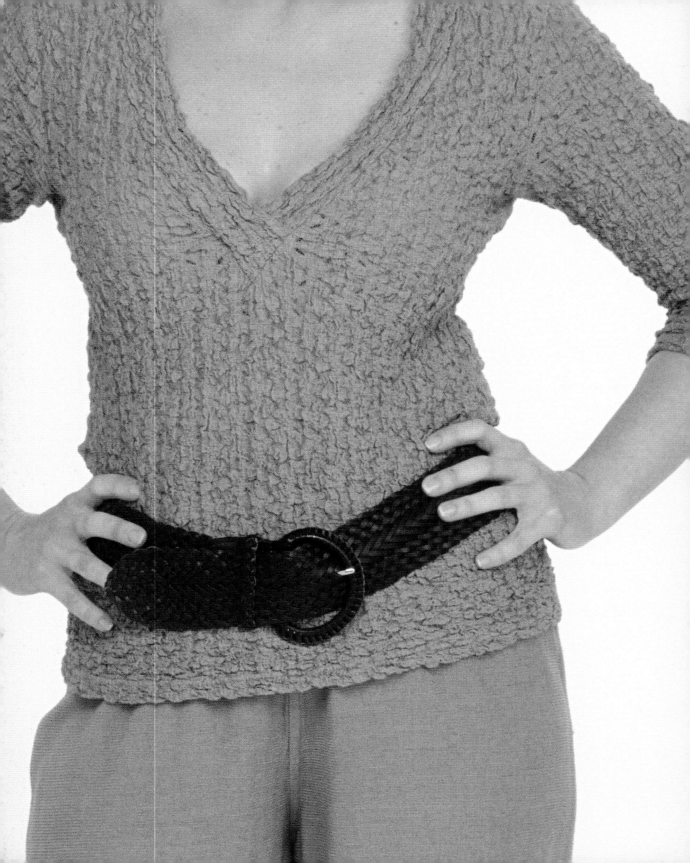

4

finding your style

Your style personality

Naturally the colour and styling of your clothes play an important part in your appearance, but it is your personality that acts as a catalyst and pulls your whole look together. Your personality dictates your style, which is your own interpretation of fashion and how you like to wear clothes.

Once you know and understand your style personality, putting your wardrobe together will become second nature. If you ignore your personality and buy clothes simply because they're featured in all the glossy magazines or look great on a friend, you will not look comfortable and your wardrobe will be a muddle of styles. This, in turn, will limit your flexibility in mixing and matching to create the perfect outfits for you. It also means that you won't get the best value from your clothing investments.

The clothes that you wear and how you wear them are governed by many factors: age, build, lifestyle, environment, budget, culture and personal preferences. The way you project yourself may be influenced by your upbringing, the way you want others to see you or even by a misguided approach to how you see yourself. Knowing your style personality will give you the foundation on which to project yourself in a more organized way, and to feel comfortable in your outfit, whatever the occasion.

Styles of the famous

Before working out your own style personality, have a look at how famous people dress. Notice what they are wearing when they appear at their most comfortable and relaxed.

Singer Gwen Stefani is a true **Creative**, changing her look constantly to suit her latest record or video. A trendsetter rather than a trend follower, she loves avant-garde designers.

Television celebrity Sharon Osbourne has a **Dramatic** style personality, choosing clothes that get her noticed and sometimes even shock. She loves setting trends and working with the latest designers to create a look that's new and different.

With her wonderful, long wavy hair, actress Nicole Kidman epitomizes the **Romantic** style personality. Away from the red carpet, she loves pretty, feminine details and luxury fabrics.

Condoleezza Rice, US Secretary of State, is an example of the **Classic** style personality. Her look is the same every time she is seen in public: simple and groomed. Nothing is out of place, nothing shocks, and she is completely co-ordinated.

Dame Ellen MacArthur, yachtswoman, has a **Natural** style personality. She doesn't care about the world seeing her unkempt, with messy hair and without any make-up.

Actress Catherine Deneuve has developed an elegance that is fashionable but not trendy. Her clothes are understated and her accessories always in vogue. It's difficult to recall exactly what she wears – you just remember that she looks good, and this is the key factor of a **City Chic** style personality.

Changing your style

As you progress though life, you will feel different about the way you look. What you wear in your early twenties, for example, will be very different from how you will want to dress when middle-aged.

In your teens you might flaunt your body by wearing revealing outfits, or follow fashion fads regardless of whether they suit you. You might

> **Knowing your style personality will enable you to feel comfortable in your outfit, whatever the occasion**

find yourself going out of your way to shock others through what you wear, or you may show no interest at all in clothes and personal grooming.

As you begin to think about attracting the opposite sex, your clothes can become an extension of your sexuality. You may start to wear make-up or apply more than you used to. You may even wear really uncomfortable items of clothing simply because they help you convey how you feel inside. If you feel romantic, you may portray that emotion on the outside by wearing feminine clothes. Floral patterns may creep into your wardrobe, fabrics may become sheerer and you may wear the odd frilly number.

As you advance in your career or become a parent, you may feel that you need a more classic look, and that you should put on a 'uniform' to suit your new status in life. You start to think about making your clothes last for more than one season. Expensive investment purchases now feature in your wardrobe, and you consider how versatile an item might be before you buy it.

There are, of course, those of you who simply enjoy clothes – you're not fashion victims, but you like to look up to date. You have experimented over the years and have discovered what suits you, and probably have some basic items that form the core of your look. You enjoy shopping for accessories and special pieces to enhance your wardrobe. Through good advice or experimentation, you will have already learnt what does and what doesn't work for you.

Some of you will have been through all these various style stages, and may feel that you are stuck in a format that's comfortable but boring. Now is the time to move on and try something new.

Identifying your look

Completing the questionnaire overleaf will help you determine your style personality. Some of you will discover that you have a split style personality, and you will need to decide which one is the most appropriate for you, although it is possible to be one type for work and another for socializing.

Those of you who are really adept at planning your wardrobe might be a little of all of the personalities, depending on the occasion and how you feel at any particular time.

Bear in mind that there is also a psychological aspect to colour and the colours that you wear: ***go to pages 28–31.***

Style personality questionnaire

To find out your style personality, complete the questionnaire below, circling as many options as you wish. You may feel that some questions merit more than one answer – for example, one may describe how you dress during the week, another may reflect your appearance at weekends, and a third may describe how you would like to look. Take the plunge and discover the real you!

How do you wear colour?

- ☐ **A** Whatever I feel like on the day.
- ☐ **B** Strong, contrasting and bright shades.
- ☐ **C** Pretty pastels.
- ☐ **D** I like to be co-ordinated.
- ☐ **E** I go for simple colour combinations.
- ☐ **F** A tone-on-tone look.

What kind of shopper are you?

- ☐ **A** I love markets and vintage clothes.
- ☐ **B** I buy something if I like it.
- ☐ **C** I enjoy the whole shopping experience.
- ☐ **D** I plan my shopping trips and take a list.
- ☐ **E** I buy when I need something.
- ☐ **F** I am an investment buyer.

How would you describe your overall look?

- ☐ **A** Eclectic and sometimes wacky.
- ☐ **B** I like to make a statement and wear eye-catching pieces.
- ☐ **C** Pretty with detailed clothes that make me feel feminine.
- ☐ **D** Neat, organized and co-ordinated.
- ☐ **E** Relaxed and casual.
- ☐ **F** Simple and elegant.

What is in your working wardrobe?

- ☐ **A** Individual pieces.
- ☐ **B** Eye-catching pieces.
- ☐ **C** Pretty blouses and tops that I combine with a jacket.
- ☐ **D** Tailored suits.
- ☐ **E** Easy-to-wear separates.
- ☐ **F** Basic pieces, but dressed up with accessories.

What is in your non-working wardrobe?

- **A** My collection of vintage clothes.
- **B** My latest fashion purchase.
- **C** Pretty, feminine pieces.
- **D** Co-ordinated separates.
- **E** Jeans and comfortable tops.
- **F** Simple styles, which I accessorize.

What is in your special occasion wardrobe?

- **A** Velvet, brocade, antiques and lace.
- **B** Unusual and striking garments.
- **C** Fitted dresses with lots of detailing.
- **D** Simple and tailored dresses.
- **E** Comfortable, dressy trousers or a long skirt with a loose-fitting top.
- **F** An elegant dress or trouser suit.

What are your shoes like?

- **A** They don't co-ordinate with my outfit.
- **B** High-heeled or funky.
- **C** Pretty, with bows and details.
- **D** They match my handbag.
- **E** Comfortable.
- **F** Current.

What kind of jewellery do you like?

- **A** Unusual – I collect it.
- **B** Bold, makes a statement.
- **C** Intricate, dangly and pretty.
- **D** Simple and fine.
- **E** Minimal.
- **F** Current and noticeable.

What is your attitude to make-up?

- **A** I experiment.
- **B** I like it to be noticed.
- **C** I love it and spend time over it.
- **D** I keep to the same routine.
- **E** Minimalistic.
- **F** It complements my look.

What type of hairstyle do you have?

- **A** It changes with my mood.
- **B** It changes regularly.
- **C** Long.
- **D** Neat.
- **E** Low maintenance.
- **F** Up to date.

Once you have completed the questionnaire, count how many times you have answered A, B, etc., and see right to determine your predominant style personality. Then refer to the following pages for examples of famous people who match your style personality and for tips on how to achieve the style.

Mainly A Creative: *go to pages 144–145*
Mainly B Dramatic: *go to pages 146–147*
Mainly C Romantic: *go to pages 148–149*
Mainly D Classic: *go to pages 150–151*
Mainly E Natural: *go to pages 152–153*
Mainly F City Chic: *go to pages 154–155*

Creative

You are great at combining different items of clothing and accessories to give yourself a unique and interesting look, and you rarely throw anything out because you know you will use it at some point, even if it has to be remodelled. If you're not careful, though, your creative tendencies could result in your being inappropriately dressed for certain occasions.

Famous Creatives

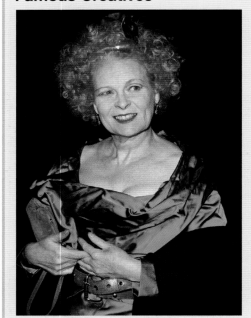

Vivienne Westwood (pictured)
Helena Bonham Carter
Sienna Miller
Kate Moss
Anita Pallenberg
Gwen Stefani

Style characteristics

✓ Your wardrobe is full of items from many different sources, including vintage mixed with high fashion, that you have collected over the years.

✓ Shopping for you is an art form. You like nothing better than rummaging around a charity shop or your mother's attic. You find chain stores distasteful.

✓ You often make interesting purchases while on holiday, and look at fashion magazines for inspiration.

Make the most of your style

✓ Team chunky knits with floaty dresses and boots.

✓ Wear trousers with tunics and dresses, teamed with a low-slung belt.

✓ Make office wear more interesting with an eye-catching blouse or a scarf, mixed with unusual accessories.

✓ For the evening, choose a vintage dress, perhaps with a pair of jewelled shoes.

Make the most of your colour palette

Light   Primrose + light aqua, geranium + blush pink, light navy + apple green.

Deep   Chocolate + aubergine, taupe + royal purple, lime + turquoise.

Warm   Tangerine + mint, purple + bittersweet, charcoal + oatmeal.

Cool   Light periwinkle + hot pink, duck egg + teal, blue-red + icy green.

Clear   Black + apple green, light apricot + royal blue, ruby + light teal.

Soft   Shell + soft violet, claret + rose brown, sage + charcoal blue.

How to accessorize

✓ Choose a belt that will make a statement.

✓ Wear a scarf that doesn't co-ordinate with or match what you are wearing.

✓ Add costume jewellery or interesting ethnic pieces as finishing touches.

✓ Customize clothes with interesting buttons.

✓ Pin a corsage or brooch to a vintage jacket to bring it up to date.

✓ Wear a hat, whatever the weather.

Your face

By day   Choose either your eyes or your lips to create a wow effect with make-up.
By night   Combine colours that do not necessarily match what you are wearing.

Your hair

Add outrageous colours to your hair. Accessorize with unusual combs, slides, flowers and scarves. Experiment with plaits and hair extensions.

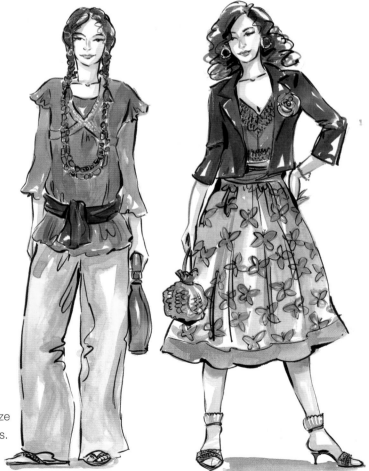

Dramatic

You always want to make an entrance. You love to be noticed and often wear clothes with a wow factor. Whatever the latest fashion, you will have a go at wearing it, even if it doesn't particularly suit you. Shopping is one of your favourite pastimes. You like to party – spending a quiet evening at home reading a book is not your scene.

Famous Dramatics

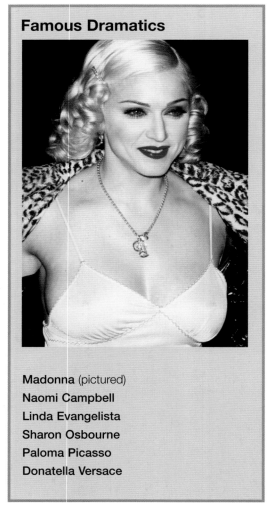

Madonna (pictured)
Naomi Campbell
Linda Evangelista
Sharon Osbourne
Paloma Picasso
Donatella Versace

Style characteristics

✓ Your wardrobe consists of many different styles of clothes and one-off pieces that you have bought on impulse, without a thought as to whether you have anything to wear with them.

✓ Your friends are often envious of your striking appearance.

✓ You are not concerned with whether your clothes are practical or washable – they must simply make a statement.

✓ You will scour the fashion press for the latest trends.

Make the most of your style

✓ Wear separates in contrasting colours.

✓ The bolder and more striking your accessories, the better.

✓ In the evening, wear that 'Oscar' dress; it's your style to dress up, rather than down, for parties and special occasions.

✓ Be prepared to tone down your look for the office.

Make the most of your colour palette

Light Light grey + geranium, peacock + blush pink, taupe + violet.

Deep Black + soft white, scarlet + damson, chocolate + fern.

Warm Purple + amber, bronze + daffodil, orange-red + aqua.

Cool Charcoal + periwinkle, cassis + royal blue, spruce + blue-green.

Clear True blue + ivory, apple green + light apricot, true red + black-brown.

Soft Purple + light periwinkle, emerald turquoise + mint, rose brown + claret.

How to accessorize

✓ Wear belts with interesting buckles and details, such as studs, jewels or cut-out patterns.

✓ Make a statement with bold patterns in contrasting colours.

✓ Wear large, striking jewellery, but not too much at once.

✓ Update your look each season with new shoes or boots.

✓ Throw a colourful scarf over your winter coat.

✓ Always wear a hat or hair accessory.

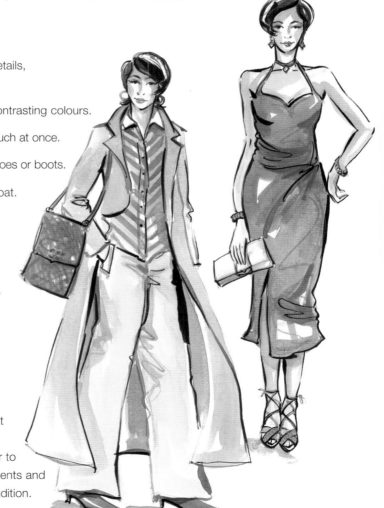

Your face

By day Don't forget your eye pencil plus two or three coats of mascara, and your lipgloss.
By night Nothing but the full works for you, finished off with a red lipstick.

Your hair

Add a striking colour to your hair (in tones that complement your colouring). Change your hairstyle regularly and consult your hairdresser to keep up with the latest styles. Use hair treatments and styling products to keep your hair in peak condition.

Romantic

You love everything about dressing up and planning your wardrobe. Your clothes are pretty and you adore all sorts of details: bows, ruffles, flounces, appliqués and fringes. You love to experiment with new skincare and bodycare products, and never go out without your perfume. You will spend longer than anybody else looking after yourself and your grooming.

Famous Romantics

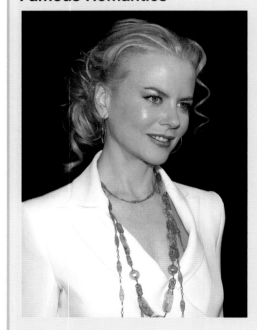

Nicole Kidman (pictured)
Sarah Ferguson, Duchess of York
Elizabeth Hurley
Scarlett Johansson
Kylie Minogue
Charlize Theron

Style characteristics

✓ Flowers feature heavily in your wardrobe, whether in patterned fabrics or as accessories and decorative details, such as corsages, brooches and other jewellery.

✓ You always wear matching and pretty underwear, even if it is uncomfortable.

✓ Your sports clothes are either in pretty colours or have decorative details.

✓ Even your business clothes are pretty and feminine.

Make the most of your style

✓ Choose separates that are decorated with beading, appliqué or ribbons.

✓ Choose luxury fabrics such as angora, cashmere, silk and satin.

✓ Skirts or dresses teamed with a cardigan or pretty jacket are a great look for you.

✓ In the evening, go for a layered look and choose fabrics such as chiffon or lace decorated with sequins and diamanté. Complete the look with high-heeled sandals.

Make the most of your colour palette

Light Light navy + pastel pink, pewter + mint, light aqua + light apricot.

Deep Charcoal + blush pink, cornflower + primrose, aubergine + moss.

Warm Coral + cream, grey-green + teal, amber + taupe.

Cool Rose pink + baby pink, sky blue + medium grey, bright periwinkle + icy green.

Clear Emerald turquoise + duck egg, scarlet + light grey, royal blue + light apricot.

Soft Blush pink + soft violet, spruce + mint, cocoa + shell.

How to accessorize

✓ Add a flower somewhere: in your hair, on your shoulder, to your bag or even your shoes.

✓ Floral prints work well if you have soft body lines; if you don't, choose spots or squiggles.

✓ Wear dangling, detailed jewellery.

✓ Decorative handbags are perfect for you.

✓ Wear fine patterned or textured tights; seamed stockings are fun if you have shapely legs.

✓ Always wear a heel, whether on a sandal or boot.

Your face

By day You always wear make-up, especially a pink lipstick and a blusher from your palette.
By night For an ultra-feminine look, dazzle with sparkle, shimmer and glitter.

Your hair

The best hairstyles for you are long and layered, softly curled and probably highlighted. Put decorations in you hair if your wear it up.

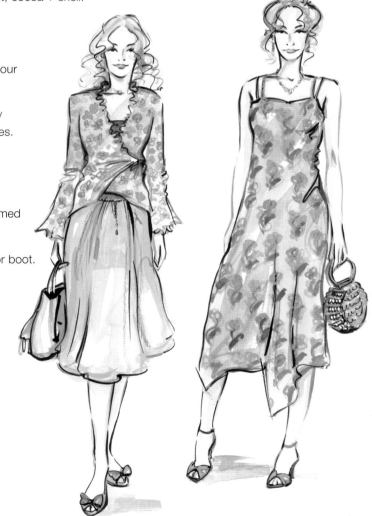

Classic

You have a fairly formal wardrobe. You like to appear well turned-out and elegant, and your tops are usually tucked in. You are quite content to keep to the same hairstyles, and hate it when your hairdresser moves away. Your make-up routine is fixed and you rarely experiment with new shades. You have a few favourite stores that you visit when you need new clothes.

Famous Classics

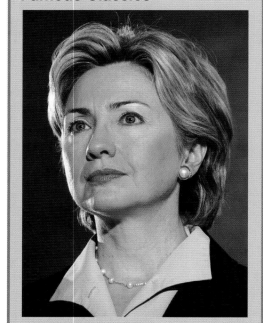

Hillary Clinton (pictured)
Laura Bush
Martina Navratilova
Princess Anne
Condoleezza Rice
Martha Stewart

Style characteristics

✓ Your look is timeless and elegant.

✓ You prefer a co-ordinated look and do not like to mix textures or wear daring colour combinations.

✓ Your work wear is smart and understated; you only ever wear pattern on scarves.

✓ At weekends you are likely to replace your jacket and blouse with a twin-set.

✓ You rarely wear jeans, preferring a smart pair of classic trousers teamed with leather loafers.

✗ You do not follow fashion.

Make the most of your style

✓ Co-ordinated separates are the basis of your look.

✓ By mixing and matching what you already have you will create many more outfits.

✓ Add coloured tops to your basic jackets to achieve a more varied look.

✓ Your evening wear will be simple, to which you will add your favourite pieces of jewellery.

Make the most of your colour palette

Light Stone + cornflower, light navy + dusty rose, cocoa + light aqua.

Deep Charcoal + burgundy, black-brown + moss, pewter + teal.

Warm Grey-green + oatmeal, chocolate + cream, bronze + amber.

Cool Dark navy + icy blue, pine + light teal, medium grey + rose pink.

Clear Black + duck egg, dark navy + emerald turquoise, taupe + blush pink.

Soft Natural beige + verbena, charcoal blue + shell, chocolate + mint.

How to accessorize

✓ Match your belt, handbag and shoes.

✓ A scarf will always finish your look.

✓ Add quality costume jewellery to the real thing to create a more varied look.

✓ The quickest way for you to update your look is with a new pair of shoes in the latest style.

✓ Change your handbag regularly.

✗ Do not wear all your favourite pieces of matching jewellery at the same time.

Your face

By day Don't be afraid to try some new eye shadow and lipstick colours once in a while.
By night Go one tone darker within your colours.

Your hair

Consider changing your hairstyle every two or three years, keeping your colour as close to your natural shade as possible. Your preferred styles are easy to manage without complicated styling techniques.

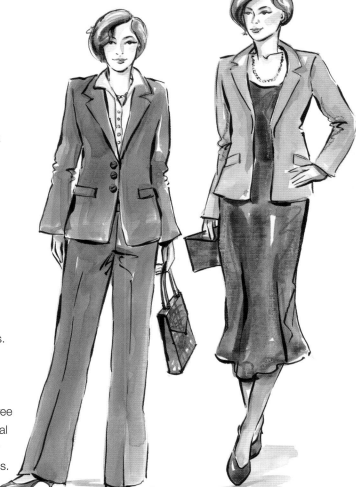

Natural

Feeling comfortable in your clothes is the most important factor for you when choosing what to wear; anything that constricts, digs in or pinches is not an option. You prefer casual styling to formal business wear, and you hate a cluttered look – simple lines and designs are more you. In keeping with your no-fuss attitude, clothes must be easy-care and ideally non-iron.

Famous Naturals

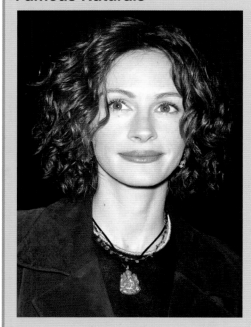

Julia Roberts (pictured)
Steffi Graf
Lauren Hutton
Sophie Marceau
Vanessa Redgrave
Kate Winslet

Style characteristics

✓ Your wardrobe may appear disorganized and you will often just wear whatever is to hand that morning.

✓ Trousers worn with flat shoes are your preferred option for maximum comfort and practicality.

✓ You have many interests but reading fashion magazines is not one of them.

✓ Your jewellery will be minimal – if you wear any at all – and won't jangle about.

Make the most of your style

✓ Long skirts – either full, pleated or with a split – will allow freedom of movement; team them with boots or comfortable shoes.

✓ Go for deconstructed and loose-fitting clothes for a relaxed look.

✓ For work, comfort is still important, so opt for a simple, good-quality top rather than a fussy, tailored shirt.

✓ For evening, try a tunic-type top over a pair of silk pants with flat pumps.

Make the most of your colour palette

Light   Stone + cornflower, medium grey + dusty rose, light navy + light aqua.

Deep   Black + aubergine, dark navy + purple, stone + true red.

Warm   Dark brown + terracotta, moss + cream, teal + turquoise.

Cool   Rose beige + sapphire, pewter + bright periwinkle, pine + light grey.

Clear   Black + evergreen, purple + lemon yellow, taupe + Chinese blue.

Soft   Stone + claret, cocoa + jade, damson + shell.

How to accessorize

✓ Your accessories will be minimal, but you still need them to complete your look.

✓ Wear a long scarf or pashmina over your coat or jacket, teamed with a pair of gloves.

✓ For jewellery, choose natural materials such as wood, leather and shell.

✓ A rucksack-style handbag or one with a long shoulder strap is best for you.

Your face

By day Your make-up is minimal, so all-in-one products like tinted moisturiser are ideal.
By night You don't tend to change your make-up dramatically for the evening; simply add a fresh slick of a natural-coloured lipstick or gloss.

Your hair

You don't like to spend much time on your tresses, so it's essential to have a good haircut that allows you to leave your hair to dry with little or no styling.

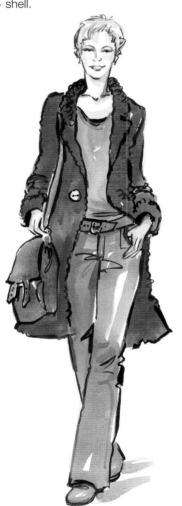
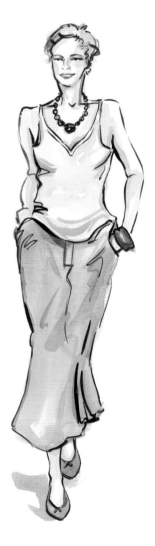

City chic

You enjoy your clothes but are not fanatical about them. You dedicate time and thought to the way you look, and you love accessories, sometimes spending more on bags and shoes than on an outfit itself. Having probably tried out most of the other key styles and experimented with lots of different looks, you now know what suits you.

Famous City Chics

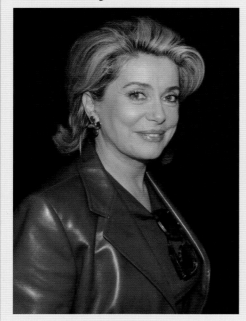

Catherine Deneuve (pictured)
Emmanuelle Béart
Honor Blackman
Isabella Rossellini
Sharon Stone
Oprah Winfrey

Style characteristics

✓ You tend to follow trends rather than high fashion.

✓ You shop with care and rarely make rash purchases, ensuring that whatever you buy co-ordinates with other items that you already have in your wardrobe.

✓ You use bright colours with caution and tend to go for a tone-on-tone look.

✓ You keep abreast of the latest trends by reading magazines.

Make the most of your style

✓ Invest in basic, classic pieces in neutral colours.

✓ Keep your working wardrobe updated with new tops, purchased regularly.

✓ Team trousers with a stylish shirt or twin-set and accessorize appropriately.

✓ For evening, a simple shift dress with a stunning necklace, worn with a colourful wrap or pashmina, will be a great success. Mules would be a good choice for footwear to complete this simple but stylish outfit.

Make the most of your colour palette

Light   Stone + cocoa, light periwinkle + sky blue, pastel pink + dusty rose.

Deep   Black + charcoal, pine + mist, purple + damson.

Warm   Bronze + moss, bittersweet + terracotta, daffodil + amber.

Cool   Medium grey + light grey, light periwinkle + dark periwinkle, cassis + rose pink.

Clear   True blue + royal blue, evergreen + emerald green, pewter + light teal.

Soft   Cocoa + rose brown, sage + spruce, damson + soft violet.

How to accessorize

✓ Make a statement with a single accessory, be it a stunning necklace, brooch or beaded scarf.

✓ Even when it's not sunny, always wear your sunglasses somewhere, such as on your head.

✓ Swap the black handbag for a colourful one.

✓ Tie a scarf to your handbag,

✓ Wear a quality watch.

✓ Wear an elegant heeled pump shoe with trousers.

Your face

By day Create a matt finish for your face, and add a touch of bronzer and a neutral lipstick.
By night Enhance your eye make-up with a granite or brown pencil and add a little sheen to your eyelids; enhance your lips with a darker shade.

Your hair

Keep your hair in good condition and have it cut regularly. Subtle highlights and lowlights will ensure a natural look.

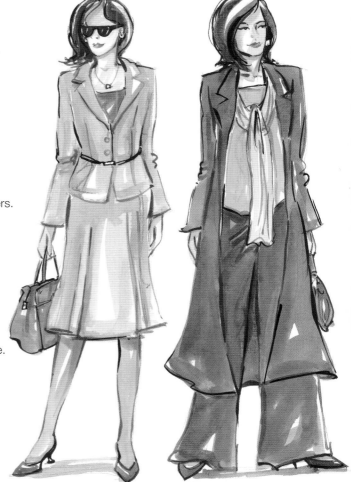

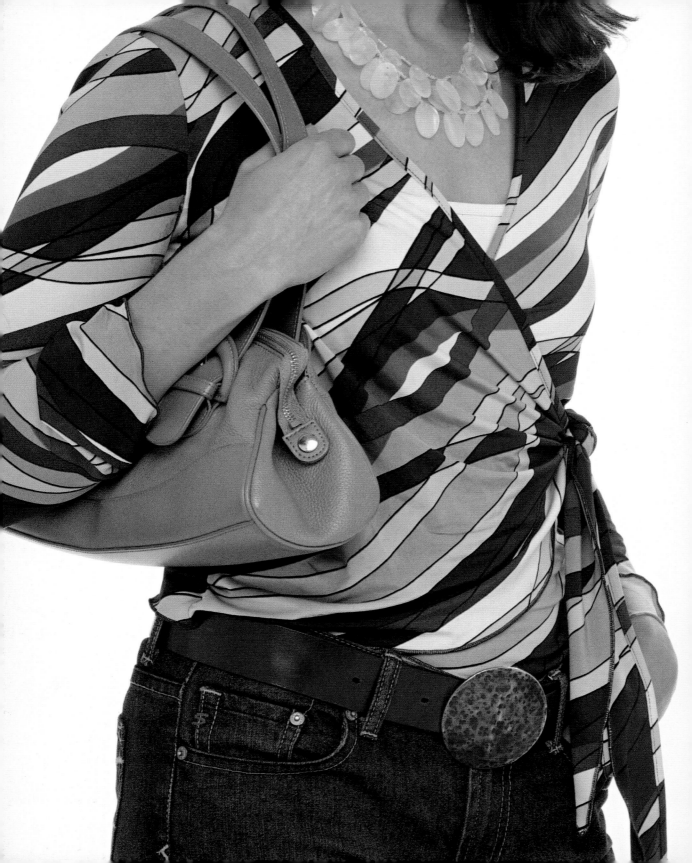

5

pulling it all together

Face shape and proportion

Now you know what clothes to wear to best complement your colouring, shape, size and style, here's how to add the finishing touches to your outfit. This chapter covers all those aspects you need to consider to pull together a complete look, from your hairstyle and make-up to your shoes, and everything in between.

Discover your face shape

Even if you have a great figure and fabulous clothes, you won't look good if your hairstyle or spectacles don't work, your underwear is wrong, or your accessories ruin the outfit.

The first step is to discover your face shape. This will help you make informed choices about your hairstyle, make-up, spectacles and earrings.

The face is divided into three sections that should be evenly proportioned:
Forehead to bridge of nose
Bridge of nose to base of nose
Base of nose to chin
The optimum face shape is oval. This means:
The widest point is at the cheekbones
The face narrows gradually down to the jaw

Step 1 – Face shape

✓ Tie or pin your hair back off your face.

✓ Wear a low neckline.

✓ Stand in front of a mirror.

✓ Using a water-soluble marker pen, draw the outline of your face onto the mirror.

✓ Stand back and look at the result.

✓ Is your basic face shape oval or round?

✓ Does your face have angles?

✓ Is the overall shape balanced?

✓ Does your face seem long?

✓ Is it wide at the top, narrowing down to a pointed chin?

Step 2 – Proportions

✓ Standing in your original position, look at the outline of your face drawn onto the mirror; mark the position of the bridge of your nose.

✓ Then draw another line at the base of your nose, and check the proportions (see above).

Step 3 – Profile

✓ Turn to the side and look at your facial profile.

✓ Is there any feature that stands out disproportionately, such as your forehead, nose or chin?

If your face shape and proportions are balanced, and you're happy with your profile, go straight to the page relating to your face shape. If not, read on.

The challenges – Proportions

High or low forehead

The best way to minimize a high forehead is with a fringe, whether full, layered or asymmetric. If you have a low forehead, wear your hair off your face; if your hair naturally grows forward, ask your hairdresser to cut a fringe from the top of your head – this is known as a deep fringe – to give the illusion of a higher forehead.

Long nose

Use make-up to help create the illusion of a shorter nose. Highlight the nostril area with a light shade of foundation or concealer, and use a darker shade down the centre of the nose. This will make the nose appear wider and shorter. Avoid a hairstyle with a centre parting.

Long chin

Make-up can also help create the illusion of a shorter chin. Apply a darker foundation or concealer to the chin area, and use a lighter shade along the cheekbones to draw attention away from the chin.

The challenges – Profile

Large nose

Apply a darker shade of foundation over the nose, and highlight the cheekbones with a lighter shade of foundation or concealer. Balance your profile with a hairstyle that adds volume to the back of your head – a hairstyle that is flat at the back will emphasize a large nose.

Double chin

Use a darker powder, such as a bronzer, to cover the offending area (foundation will rub off on your clothes). To draw the eye away from the chin, emphasize your eyes or lips by using slightly brighter make-up. Anything around the neck, such as a high neckline, choker-type necklace or scarf tied high, will draw attention to a double chin, so opt for open necklines, longer necklaces and loosely tied scarves.

Ears that stick out

Don't wear your hair tucked behind or cut around your ears – you need volume around and behind them. Avoid earrings that make a statement as these will draw attention to your ears.

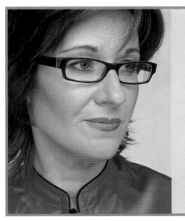

How to choose spectacles

When you are choosing spectacles, you need to take into account your dominant colour characteristics and your style personality, as well as considering your face shape and proportions. Check where the spectacles sit on your nose: if you have a long nose the bridge of the spectacles should sit lower down to make your nose seem shorter; if you have a short nose the bridge should sit higher. Your eyes should be in the centre of the lenses. For more advice on spectacles, see the relevant face shape: *go to pages 160–164*.

Oval

A balanced, oval face is the most versatile face shape and gives you many options for hairstyles, make-up, spectacles and earrings, since lots of styles will suit you. Yours is the face shape that everyone wants to have.

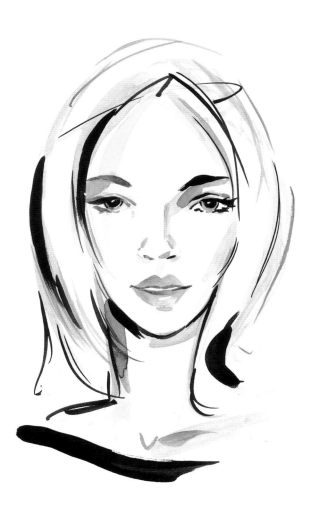

Make-up

Eyebrows Shape them so that they slant slightly upwards at the end.
Eye shadow Use eye pencil and shadow to create an almond-shaped eye: *go to page 170*.
Blusher Follow the natural line of your cheekbones, sweeping the brush upwards and outwards towards the hairline.
Lipstick As long as your upper and lower lips are balanced, follow your natural lip line.
Top tip Apply a hint of blusher to the tip of the chin and around the temples.

Hairstyle

Any style will complement an oval face shape, but take into account your neck length, age and hair type. If you feel confident, wear your hair completely swept away from your face.

Spectacles

Most shapes and styles will suit you, except extreme geometric designs.

Earrings

If you have a short neck, you should avoid long, chandelier-type earrings. Otherwise, you can wear any style.

For more advice on applying make-up:
go to pages 165–173.

Square

You have a wide forehead, and your cheekbones are in line with your jaw. To create a more balanced face shape, you can use clever shading to soften the squareness of your jaw and emphasize your cheekbones.

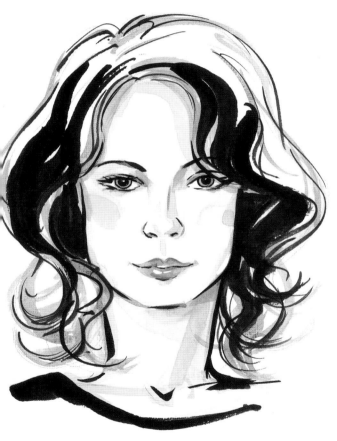

Make-up

Eyebrows Shape your eyebrows to create a gentle arch above the centre of each eye, directly over the pupil.

Eye shadow Apply highlighter under the centre of the eyebrow and blend eye shadow, using upward strokes, towards the outer edge of the eye.

Blusher Apply blusher in a gently curved line along the cheekbones.

Lipstick Use a lip pencil to make your lips slightly fuller in the middle.

Top tip Apply darker shading (bronzer) on the edge of your jawline to soften the angle.

Hairstyle

Aim to add width to the upper part of your face, and soften the angles with curls or layers. Avoid straight bobs and heavy, straight fringes.

Spectacles

Look for lightweight oval or rounded styles. Avoid square or rectangle shapes which will emphasize the angles of your face.

Earrings

Rounded shapes, such as hoops and ovals, are best; avoid sharp or angular designs.

For more advice on applying make-up: *go to pages 165–173*.

Rectangle

You have a long, narrow face with a squarish chin. You need to give the illusion of widening and shortening the face, while softening the jawline. Horizontal lines make the face look wider, so emphasize your eyebrows, cheekbones and lips.

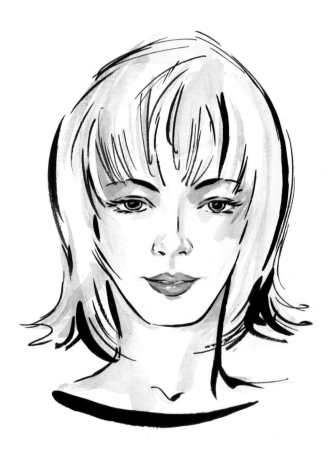

Make-up

Eyebrows Use a brow pencil to slightly extend the outer tails of your eyebrows, adding width.
Eye shadow Layer toning colours horizontally, working from the centre of the eye outwards.
Blusher Follow the lines of your cheekbones, adding more definition near the hairline.
Lipstick Make your mouth look slightly wider when you line your lips, but keep it looking natural.
Top tip Apply a sweep of blusher along the hairline at cheekbone level to draw the eye outwards.

Hairstyle

A layered style will help give the impression that your face is rounder and fuller. A softly layered crown is good, as is some fullness around the ear area. A fringe will also make your face appear shorter. Avoid long, straight styles with a centre parting, as these will make your face look longer.

Spectacles

Lightweight, wider frames will counteract a narrow face and close-set eyes; avoid angular frames.

Earrings

Choose curvy shapes that add volume to your earlobes. Avoid long, dangly styles.

For more advice on applying make-up: *go to pages 165–173*.

Inverted triangle

You have a broad forehead and cheekbones, which taper down to a small chin. Aim to give the illusion of a narrower brow and cheekbones by adding volume and interest to your jawline.

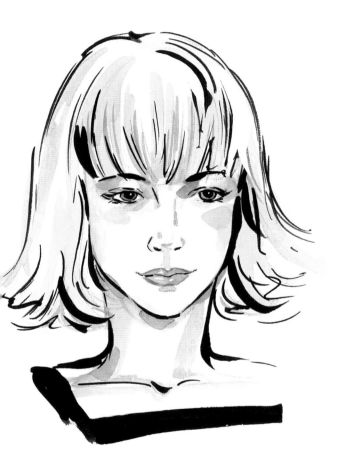

For more advice on applying make-up:
go to pages 165–173.

Make-up

Eyebrows Slightly shorten the natural length of your eyebrows and shape them into a gentle arch.
Eye shadow Highlight the centre of the eyelid and create a rounded shape on the outer corners.
Blusher Apply only to the apples of the cheeks.
Lipstick Make your mouth appear wider using liner, and fill in the colour right to the edge.
Top tip Lipglosses and sheens are a must.

Hairstyle

Your hairstyle should add volume and interest to your jawline. A one-length bob that finishes just below your earlobe and which is turned in or flipped out is ideal. Pulled-back styles or styles that add volume around the temples are not for you; a fringe should be light and feathered.

Spectacles

The frames should not extend beyond your temples. Frameless spectacles are an excellent choice, and the arms should be lightweight.

Earrings

Choose large earrings that will draw attention to your jawline. Dangly styles are great if you have a long neck.

Round

Although the softness of a round face can be attractive, creating angles and vertical lines through your choice of hairstyle and clever application of make-up will help give the illusion of a more balanced face shape.

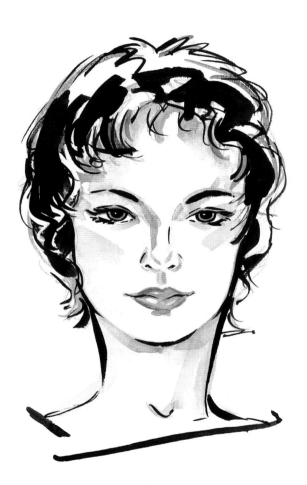

For more advice on applying make-up:
go to pages 165–173.

Make-up

Eyebrows Keep your eyebrows as straight as possible and don't let the outer corner droop.
Eye shadow Apply colours in diagonal lines that slant up towards the outer corners of your eyes.
Blusher Apply blusher in a straight line along the cheekbones.
Lipstick Create a wider, slightly narrower mouth when lining your lips.
Top tip Use a highlighter (or shine or gloss) along the top of the cheekbone to create angles.

Hairstyle

Asymmetric partings and fringes are flattering, while a light, feathered style will break up the fullness of the face. Avoid a big bubbly perm, or a rounded bob that frames the face.

Spectacles

Frames that are slightly wider than your face will make your face seem smaller. Square or rectangular frames balance a round face, but avoid round shapes and full, frameless lenses.

Earrings

Choose angled or dangly styles (if you have a long neck), but avoid round or hooped earrings.

Make-up know-how

You don't have to spend hours in front of the mirror every day, but you deserve to look your best at all times. After all, research has shown that women who wear make-up look younger, earn more and get promoted more quickly. The following advice has helped thousands of women achieve a polished and groomed look without being overly made-up.

As well as giving you a well-groomed, polished appearance, make-up can work magic. By placing lines and colours in the correct places, you can 'adjust' the proportions of your face to create a more balanced face shape, giving the illusion of a smaller nose, bigger eyes or a smaller chin, for example.

Remember these principles:

Light colours highlight and draw attention
Dark colours make things look smaller
Soft and muted colours minimize
Bright and clear colours emphasize

Tool kit

For the most successful results, you need to use the correct make-up tools. Treat yourself to some good-quality brushes. Natural bristle brushes are the preferred choice of make-up artists, as they are gentler on the skin and shed less than synthetic brushes. Keep them in good condition by washing them once a week in mild shampoo; rinse well, blot, then stand them upright to dry. Storing your kit in one place – in the bathroom or on a dressing table – will help speed up your routine. Below are the key items you will need.

Lip brush (1)
Concealer brush (2)
Angled eye shadow brush (3)
Blender brush (4)
Blusher brush (5)

Cosmetic sponge
Powder brush
Eyelash curlers
Pencil sharpener
Cotton-wool pads
Cotton buds (Q-tips)

Application techniques

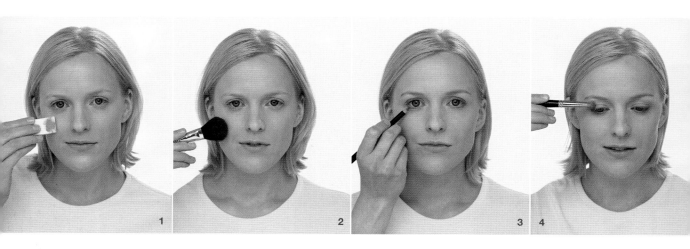

These basic make-up application techniques and tips will help you to achieve professional results. You can adapt the steps depending on how long you want to spend on your make-up, and on the occasion. For example, for a day at work you may want nothing more than a light base, such as a tinted moisturizer, and a slick of mascara. For a special night out, though, you may want to emphasize your eyes more than usual with eyeliner and several shades of eye shadow, or play up your lips. Whatever your routine, whether you wear a lot or little make-up, always start with a clean and freshly moisturized face.

Step 1 – Foundation

First of all, use a skin adjuster to camouflage any blemishes, broken veins or dark circles under the eyes. Most skin adjusters come in two shades: green to counteract red blemishes; yellow to counteract dark shadows and pink blemishes.

Apply foundation or tinted moisturizer, using either a cosmetic sponge or your fingertips and working on one part of the face at a time. Avoid your eyelids and lips, and do not dot the foundation over your nose, forehead, cheeks and chin – it will dry as it contacts the air and result in uneven coverage. Finally, apply concealer to hide any visible blemishes.

Step 2 – Powder

To set your make-up, apply loose powder to the bony areas of your face with a cotton-wool pad to press the powder in. Use downward strokes with your powder brush to remove excess powder.

Step 3 – Eyeliner

Using an appropriate shade of eye pencil, line the outer third of the lower lid, and the outer two-thirds of the upper lid.

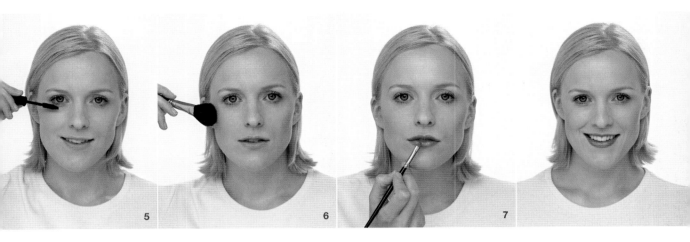

Step 4 – Eye shadow

Apply an eye base evenly all over the eyelids to fix your eye shadow and prevent it from creasing. Following the guidelines for your particular eye shape (page 170), use a blender brush to apply highlighter or a light or neutral shade of eye shadow from the lashes to the eyebrow. Then add a dark, neutral or accent eye shadow along the lower third of the eyelid and blend. You can use up to four shades of eye shadow if desired.

Step 5 – Brows and lashes

Brush your eyebrows against the direction of growth, then brush them back into shape. If necessary, use an eyebrow pencil to lengthen and correct the shape and colour (pages 160–164). Curled lashes open up the eye; start close to the roots and work towards the tips maintaining even pressure. Apply one to two coats of mascara to your top and bottom lashes, concentrating on the tips. Separate the lashes using an eyelash comb before the mascara dries.

Step 6 – Blusher

Apply blusher along the cheekbones, following the guidelines relating to your face shape (pages 160–164) and building up the colour gradually to the desired depth. Powder blush should be applied with a brush, while cream blusher, which is more forgiving on older skin, can be applied with a brush or fingertips.

Step 7 – Lips

Apply lip base to make your lipstick last longer. Follow the guidelines for your particular lip shape (page 171). Outline your lips with a pencil and fill in for more depth of colour. Apply lipstick, blot, then reapply and finish with lip gloss if desired.

Evening glamour

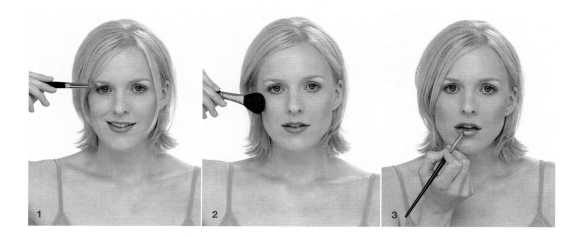

Sometimes, it calls for a little magic at the end of a hectic day to transform you. Even if you don't have time to start from scratch, these tips will help take you from daytime beauty to evening belle. Refer to the techniques on the previous pages, but note that your face needs more colour in artificial light, so choose stronger shades for eyes and lips. Remove your make-up (leave your eye make-up intact if you don't have much time). Apply moisturizer, then reapply your foundation, concealer and powder.

Step 1 – The eyes

Use a darker shade of eye pencil and a brighter accent eye shadow (or one with a sheen). A dash of gold or silver powder on the centre of both eyelids will make your eyes sparkle. Reapply your mascara, emphasizing the outer edges of the eyes to give a wide-eyed expression. Reapply your eyebrow colour if necessary.

Step 2 – The cheeks

Choose a deeper shade of blusher from your palette to give your cheeks more colour and definition. Apply blusher to the apple of your cheek, working upwards and outwards.

Step 3 – The lips

Choose either the darkest or brightest lipstick colour from your palette. Apply lip base for more staying power, then line and fill in your lips with a toning lip liner. Apply lipstick as before, then add a coat of gloss for extra sheen.

Step 4 – Finishing touches

Using a large powder brush, sweep bronzing powder over the prominent parts of your face (temple, cheekbones, chin and tip of nose). Don't forget a splash of perfume.

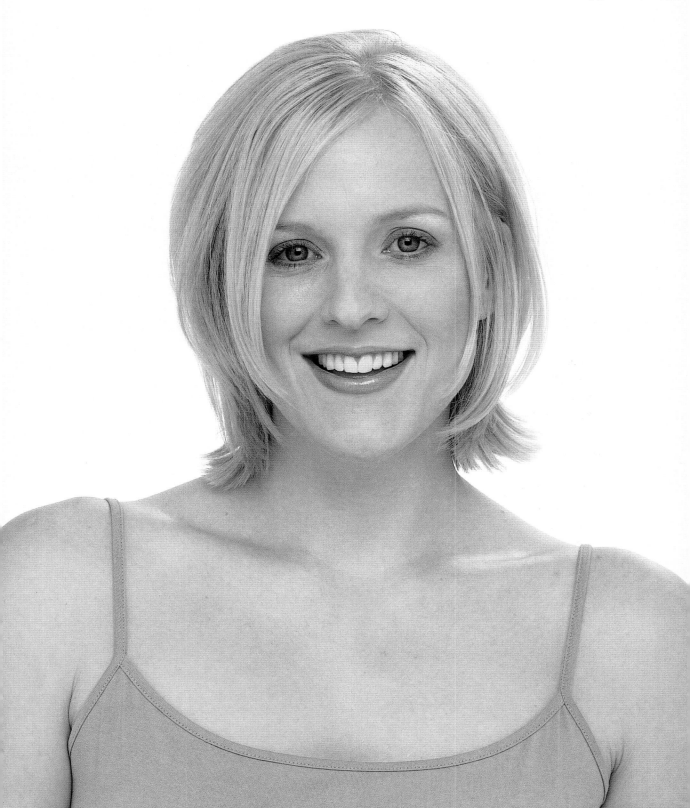

The eyes have it

Eyes come in all shapes and sizes – close-set, deep-set, slanting, and with small or large lids. As with different face shapes, there are various make-up tricks you can employ to balance the shape of your eyes and show them off to their best advantage. The most common problems and solutions are given below.

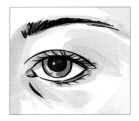

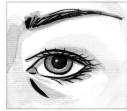

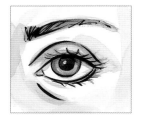

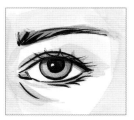

Proportioned or almond-shaped eyes

- Two-thirds of the eye area is brow and one-third is lid.
- Using a blender brush, apply highlighter from lashes to brow.
- Line the outer two-thirds of the top lid and one third of the lower lid with pencil.
- Using an angled brush apply a neutral shade of eye shadow along the orbital bone.
- Apply an accent colour to the upper lid, ending in a triangle at the outer corner.
- Finally, apply neutral eye shadow to blend the colours together.

Small lids, large brow area

- Balance the eye by creating a natural contour on the brow area and light colours on the eyelids.
- With a blender brush, apply matte highlighter from lashes to brow.
- Line two-thirds of the lower lid, and one-third of the top lid.
- Use an angled brush to apply a neutral shade of eye shadow in a wide arch over the fleshiest part of the brow.
- Bracket the outer corner of the eyelid with an accent colour, then blend, but keep the eyelids light.

Prominent lids, small brow area

- The sockets may seem deep-set and the brow area narrow. Make the lids less prominent, and elongate the eyes.
- With a blender brush, apply a light or neutral shade to lids and brows.
- Line the bottom lid with a dark pencil and apply a wide line across the top lid, blending upwards and outwards at the corner.
- Apply a similar colour over the entire lid, then blend with a soft or neutral shadow.
- Apply lots of mascara to curled lashes.

Small lids, small brow area

- Shape your eyebrows to increase the eye area.
- Apply highlighter over the whole area with a blender brush.
- Line two-thirds of the bottom lid and one-third of the top lid with pencil, extending slightly beyond the outer corner.
- Apply an accent shadow close to the lashes on the top lid, winging up and out at the corner.
- Apply the same colour over the pencil on the lower lids. Use a neutral shade to blend and soften the colours.

The lips have it

The perfect pout is the crowning glory to your make-up, but it takes a little work to get it just right. Whether your mouth is full, thin, wide or small, make the most of it by following the guidelines below. Remember, filling in the lips with pencil gives definition, and you should always blot after the first coat of lipstick, then reapply.

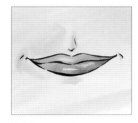 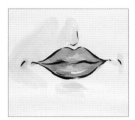 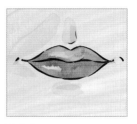 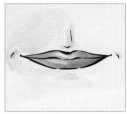

Wide mouth
● The aim is to make your mouth appear fuller and smaller.
● Apply lip pencil within the inside corner of the mouth.
● Fill in the colour, then apply two coats of lipstick.
● Apply gloss only to the centre of the lips.

Small mouth
● The aim is to give the illusion of a wider mouth.
● Apply lip pencil to extend the outer edges of the mouth, and fill in the colour.
● Use a lip brush to apply your lipstick, making sure you cover all of the new shape you have created.
● Apply gloss all over the lips.

Full lips
● The darkest shades in your palette work best. Avoid high-sheen and frosted formulations, which will make your lips look bigger.
● Apply lip pencil within the natural lip line and fill in for extra definition.
● Apply two coats of lipstick, blotting after the first coat.

Thin lips
● The lightest lipstick shades in your palette work best.
● Apply lip pencil just beyond the natural lip line and fill in the colour for definition.
● Using a lip brush, apply a coat of lipstick, blot and reapply.
● Use a sheer lipstick or gloss to highlight the centre of the lower lip.

Unbalanced lips
If one lip is fuller than the other, balance them using one light and one dark shade. On the fuller lip, apply lip pencil within the natural line of lip; on the thinner lip, apply pencil beyond the natural line. Apply a darker lipstick to the fuller lip and a lighter shade to the thinner lip.

Changing faces

Nothing dates a woman so much as wearing the same make-up at 50 as she did when she was 25 – your style of make-up and the way you apply it should change as you mature. A good skincare regime and a healthy lifestyle, together with the right clothes, colours and style, are essential for looking good and feeling confident. Here are a few winning tips to help you evolve your look.

When you are 30–40

✓ You should have established a good skincare routine: cleansing, toning and moisturizing every day; exfoliating and applying a treatment mask appropriate to your skin type – dry, oily, sensitive or normal – once a week.

✓ Ensure that you are using high-factor sunblocks all year round to protect your skin from harmful UVB rays and ageing UVA rays.

✓ Learn to recognize good-quality cosmetic products that offer the most benefits.

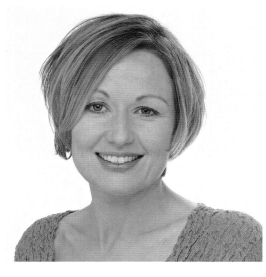

✓ Wear make-up every day to protect your skin.

✓ You are no longer a teenager, so make-up with glitter and sparkle should only be worn for parties, and even then in moderation.

✓ High-fashion make-up looks are for the catwalk only.

✓ Make regular appointments with a hygienist to ensure you have a dazzling smile.

A good skincare regime and a healthy lifestyle will keep you looking and feeling good

When you are 40–50

✓ Keep positive when the first grey hairs and lines appear.

✓ Throw away frosted eye shadows, glossy lipsticks and coloured mascaras. Don't overdo the fake tan and avoid orangey shades.

✓ Feed and nourish your skin regularly.

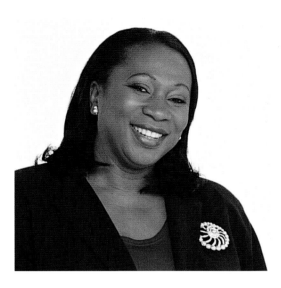

✓ Keep to a simple make-up routine, applying a minimum of base (foundation or tinted moisturizer and concealer as necessary), blusher, mascara and lipstick.

✓ Don't be afraid to use a little powder to create a more groomed look, but be careful not to apply too much and make sure you blend it well, because it can collect in and draw attention to fine lines.

✓ Use blushers and bronzers to emphasize facial bone structure and add definition to your face, particularly if you're carrying a little extra weight.

When you are 50 +

✓ Indulge yourself with the occasional pampering treat at a spa or beauty salon.

✓ A skincare regime is a must. Now is the time to use products that have been specially formulated for mature skins.

✓ Keep abreast of the latest beauty technology so that you can benefit from new products.

✓ Don't forget the rest of your body. Use a skin-firming moisturizer morning and night and always after bathing.

✓ Pay special attention to your décolletage – smooth face cream downwards and body cream upwards.

✓ Your beauty routine will now include paying more attention to your eyebrows. As well as shaping, they may need a little colour added.

✓ Less is more when it comes to make-up.

✓ An eye base is now essential, as it will prevent your lids from looking creased when wearing eye shadow.

✓ A lip base will help to prevent lipstick from bleeding and avoid a 'buttonhole' lip.

✓ Use powder on the bony parts of your face only, and avoid the soft, fleshy areas.

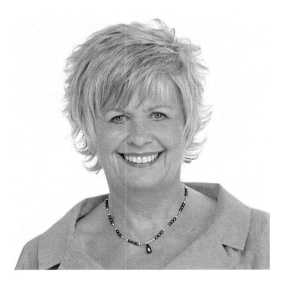

Underwear

Overdecorated underwear will show through close-fitting garments. Underwear should co-ordinate with the colours of your outer garments, and should not be seen unless you're making a fashion statement.

Bras

A bra is an important investment as it provides essential support for your breasts as well as creating the foundation for your outfit.

✓ Buy bras for different outfits and occasions: seamless, strapless, sports and so on.

✓ Get measured professionally once a year and try on a range of styles from different brands – some cuts will fit you better than others.

✓ The back of your bra should sit in the middle of your back.

✓ Your breasts should not hang over the cups.

✓ If you have heavy breasts, a bra with non-stretch straps will be more supportive.

✓ If you have a fleshy back three hooks are better than two.

✓ Fasten a new bra on the widest hooks and move inwards as the bra stretches with wear.

Knickers/Panties

There is no excuse for visible panty lines (VPLs); with so much choice available, you should be able to find a cut and fit that's right for you.

✓ Buy bigger size panties than you think you will need. This will eliminate visible panty lines by ensuring that the elastic doesn't cut into your flesh. Panties are also notorious for shrinking in the wash.

✓ If you need tummy control, make sure the fit is good and that your flesh doesn't roll over the top when you sit down.

Tights/pantyhose

A woman used not to be considered properly dressed unless she wore tights/pantyhose, whatever the weather. Nowadays, unless you work in a formal environment or are attending a formal event, it is usually acceptable to go without tights/pantyhose in summer, as long as your legs are hair- and blemish-free. However, always wear tights/pantyhose with a suit.

✓ Natural-coloured tights/pantyhose are suitable for most occasions.

✓ To elongate the legs, wear tights/pantyhose that are the same colour as your skirt or shoes.

✓ Balance the denier of your tights/pantyhose with the fabric weight of your skirt or trousers. In summer, with a lightweight fabric, seven to ten denier is ideal. In winter, with corduroy or tweed, you may consider opaques (30+ denier).

✓ Textured tights/pantyhose will give your outfit a fun twist, but they can add volume to the leg.

Accessories

Shoes and boots will update your look easily, so you should invest in at least one new pair every season. Bags and hats are also key items in creating your look and are a good way to reinforce your style personality. Belts are useful for balancing your proportions, but the style you choose and how you wear it will depend on your body shape. Scarves are a great way to introduce your colours.

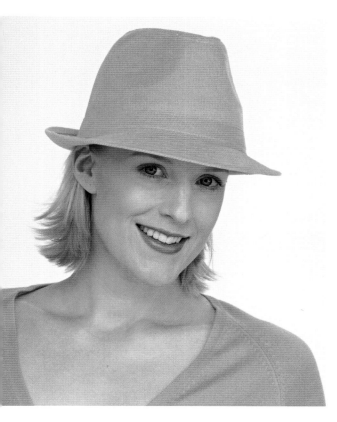

Accessories are the easiest way to introduce colour to your wardrobe

Hats

Hats date quickly and won't necessarily have much longevity in your wardrobe. However, they can turn a plain outfit into something special.

✓ Hat brims should not extend beyond your shoulders.

✓ Grand-scale women should avoid pill-box hats, which will look out of proportion.

✓ Petite women should not be tempted by large, wide-brimmed hats (picture hats).

✓ Complement your face with your hat shape. Rounded crowns, and brims in loosely woven straw or soft fabrics suit round faces.

✓ Square or rectangular faces will look good in flat crowns and straight brims, in fine straw or lightweight felt.

✓ A downward-sloping brim doesn't work with a short neck, and can emphasize jowls; a brim with an upward tilt will help to lift the face.

✓ A completely co-ordinated outfit with matching hat looks contrived; a complementary or contrasting colour adds interest to an outfit.

✓ Dark colours cast a shadow over your face.

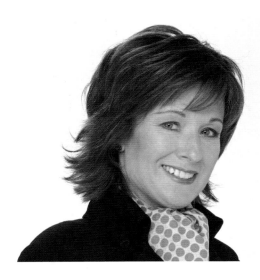

Scarves

Even if you don't own many clothes in your colours, a scarf is a great way to experiment and instantly gives you the right shade near your face.

✓ Petite women should avoid oversized scarves, such as full-size pashminas, as these can swamp you.

✓ Skinny scarves will look out of proportion on grand-scale women.

✓ Do not tie scarves under your chin if you have a short neck.

✓ A long, thin scarf draped around your neck will make your body appear taller and slimmer.

Belts

Belts are great fashion accessories that can update your look. Worn cleverly, belts can also help to balance the proportions of your upper and lower body.

✓ You need a waist to wear a belt, so they are not ideal for Lean Columns, Rectangles or Round body shapes.

✓ Narrow and lightweight belts are best on petite to average women.

✓ Wide, statement belts are best on average to grand-scale women.

✓ Belts must work with the rest of your look.

Bags

As well as carrying belongings, your handbag makes a style statement, and the bag you choose will be dictated by your style personality: *go to pages 138–155*. Like shoes, a bag can make or break your look, so here are some key pointers to help you make a choice:

✓ Different occasions call for different styles and sizes of handbag, so try to build up a collection that is appropriate for various occasions and outfits. Don't take a floral straw bag to a business meeting, nor a formal leather handbag to a dinner dance.

✓ Your bag needs to be in balance with your overall scale: a large bag will overwhelm a petite person, while a tiny bag will look lost on a grand-scale woman.

✓ The shape of your bag needs to follow the line of your body.

✓ Rectangles, Lean Columns and Inverted Triangles need structured bags to reflect the lines and angles of their bodies.

✓ Softer, unstructured bags work best for those with a Full Hourglass or Round shape.

✓ Triangles should avoid bags that hang at hip level, as they will add width to the widest area.

✓ Before you buy a handbag, look at yourself carrying it to check it looks right for you.

Footwear

Like all your accessories, the type of shoes or boots you wear can kill your look, so make sure they are appropriate for your outfit. Here are some guidelines for buying shoes and boots:

✓ The height of heel you choose will often be determined by your comfort level, but a high or a narrow heel always adds length to the leg.

✓ If you are wearing a short skirt, a lower heel will make your legs look longer.

✓ Low-fronted shoes give the illusion of longer legs and narrower ankles; closed shoes shorten the length of the feet and legs.

✓ When choosing shoes with straps, bear in mind that low-cut T-straps work for most people, while ankle straps will only look good on those with long legs and slim ankles.

✓ When buying boots, check that the boot – whether ankle, calf-height or full-length – stops at a narrow point on your legs.

✓ Sandals are ideal for holidays and hot weather, but your feet must be in immaculate condition. They should never be worn with business suits.

✓ Ballet pumps are wonderful for anyone with average to long legs and thin ankles. Satin, velvet or beaded pumps are good choices for evening, teamed with long skirts or trousers.

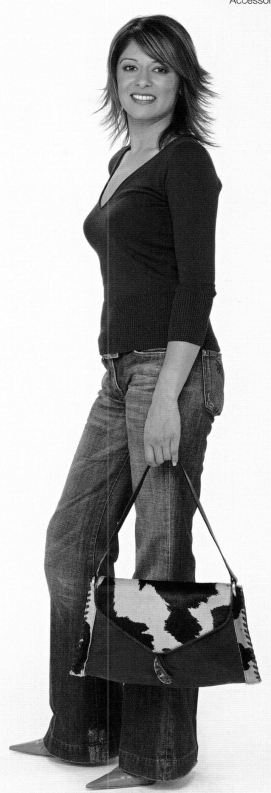

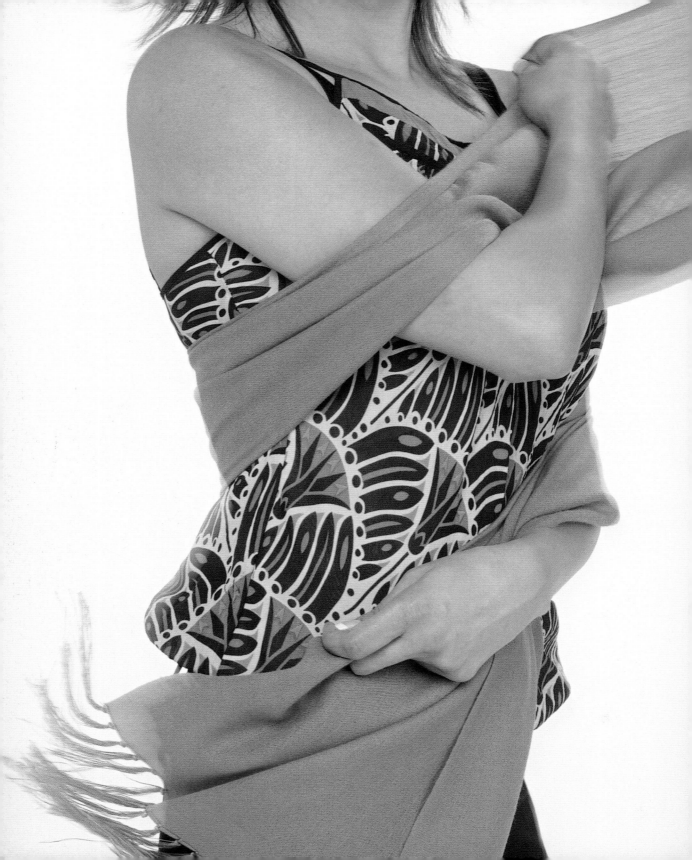

6

making your wardrobe work

Organizing your wardrobe

Now you've established your colours, style personality and body shape, and seen how to pull a look together, you have to make it all work for you. Start at the place where you keep most of your clothes: your wardrobe.

Wardrobe audit

The best way to check out what you have, what works and what doesn't work in your wardrobe is to go through each item of clothing piece by piece. Allow yourself at least a day to do this.

You will end up with three piles:
Pile 1 Clothes you will keep
Pile 2 Clothes you might keep
Pile 3 Clothes that must go

How you decide
✓ Is it the right colour? If the answer is yes, then ask yourself if it is the right style? If it is, it goes in pile 1.

✓ If it's the right colour but the wrong style, can it be altered or worn differently to make it work? If it can, it goes in pile 2.

✓ Is it the right style, but the wrong colour? Can you wear it with a complementary colour from your palette? Do you have a scarf in a colour that will make it work? If yes, it goes in pile 2.

✓ If it's the wrong colour and the wrong style, it goes in pile 3.

✓ If it's not your current size and you haven't worn it for a year, it goes in pile 3.

Pile 1 – Clothes for keeps

✓ Organize garments by categories: coats, jackets, suits, skirts, trousers, dresses, blouses and shirts. Grouping by colour within these categories will give you ideas for combining clothes.

✓ Button up jackets and coats, and pull up zips, so that garments hang straight before you put them in the wardrobe, all facing the same way.

✗ Don't put anything back in the wardrobe unless it's clean.

✗ Don't overcrowd your wardrobe.

Pile 2 – Is it worth keeping?

✓ Check every piece against what you have in your wardrobe to see whether it is worth keeping. You might find that a jacket in the wrong colour, for example, can be made to work for you if worn with a top that you've decided to keep.

✓ Shortening the hem will salvage a skirt that's too long.

✓ Changing the buttons on a jacket will give it a new lease of life.

Pile 3 – Dispose of clothes as you see fit

✓ Give them to a friend.

✓ Sell expensive items and those that are still current and of good quality.

✓ Donate them to a charity shop.

Finishing touches

Before you put everything back in your wardrobe, vacuum and dust it, and perhaps place some moth-repellent products at the bottom. To preserve the shape of your clothes, you will need the correct hangers.

✓ Sturdy wooden hangers for jackets and coats.

✓ Wooden hangers with clips for skirts and trousers.

✓ Padded hangers for lightweight and luxury fabrics.

✓ Basic plastic hangers for blouses, shirts and lightweight summer dresses.

How to shop

Inevitably, in the course of organizing your wardrobe, you will dispose of items that need to be replaced in colours and styles that suit you. To help you in this next phase, make a list of what you need to complete your wardrobe.

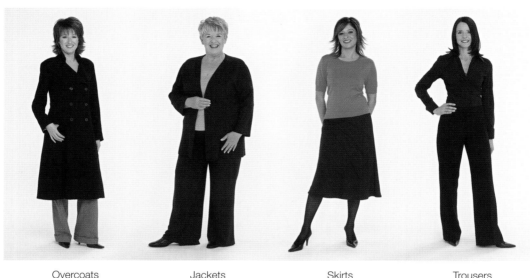

Overcoats   Jackets   Skirts   Trousers

Investment pieces should form the core of your wardrobe

Investment buys

It's not the cost of an investment buy that matters, it's how often you wear it. A bargain garment that you wear only once is a costly purchase compared to an expensive item that you wear a hundred times. Investment pieces will vary according to your lifestyle and personality, but they will generally consist of **overcoats, jackets, skirts** and **trousers.**

Fashion buys

These are the items that you buy every year to keep your core wardrobe updated and that are fun to wear. It could be anything from a current colour or the latest style in tops or dresses.

It's the fit that counts

✓ Sizes will vary depending on where you shop and the cut of the item.

✓ The looser the fit, the slimmer you look – and you'll undoubtedly feel more comfortable.

Achieving an elegantly loose fit

✓ You should be able to fit a finger underneath a waistband.

✓ Side seams should hang straight with no horizontal creases.

✓ Zips should lie flat.

✓ Allow some give in the sleeve around the upper arm.

✓ Skirts and trousers should hang straight from the buttocks and not curve under.

✓ Sleeves on jackets and coats should finish at the wrist.

✗ Pockets shouldn't gape.

✗ There should be no pulling around the bust on jackets, blouses or dresses.

Recognizing quality

✓ Seams should lie flat and not pull or wrinkle.

✓ Hemlines should be flat and even.

✓ Linings or facings must lie flat and not show.

✗ An expensive price tag doesn't always mean a quality finish.

✗ Buttonholes should not have loose threads.

Shopping tips

✓ Make a list but don't be overambitious about how much you can achieve in one trip.

✓ Wear appropriate underwear.

✓ Take with you the shoes that you'll be wearing with the garment you're buying.

✓ Look first for the right colour: *go to pages 34–105*; then ensure the style suits your body shape, proportion and scale: *go to pages 106–137*; and, finally, your style personality: *go to pages 138–155*.

✓ Take only three or four pieces at a time into the changing room.

✓ Make sure the item fits and feels comfortable.

✓ Do you like yourself in it?

✓ If it's over your budget, is it really worth it?

✓ Beware the overenthusiastic sales assistant.

Keeping it looking good

✓ Clothes that crease easily, such as linens, need laundering after each wearing; tailored suits need to be hung up in order for them to air.

✓ Shoes absorb moisture when they're worn, which needs to evaporate before you wear them again.

✓ Keep dry-cleaning to a minimum, as the fluids will damage and weaken the fibres.

✓ Repair any damage to your clothes (loose hems, missing buttons or snags) immediately.

✓ Clean shoes regularly, and use shoe trees.

Formal capsule

You don't need a wardrobe full of clothes to be well dressed for work and formal situations. By developing a 'capsule' wardrobe of basic pieces that you can mix and match, you can be confident of looking your best whatever the occasion.

Main wardrobe

Suits/jackets, skirts and trousers
Four suits in complementary neutral colours, or a combination of four jackets and four skirts or pairs of trousers.

Tops
Six to eight tops, shirts or knitwear items in your colours. Tops are a good way of introducing colour to your wardrobe – if you choose white for the majority of your tops, you'll look the same every day.

Dresses
You can wear dresses instead of skirts and tops.

Overcoat
One coat or raincoat that will fit over your suit.

Accessories

Shoes
Three pairs of formal shoes that fit with current trends and are appropriate to the season.

Bags
Two quality handbags, in appropriate colours. If you're using them for work, make sure they're large enough to hold documents and folders. Avoid struggling with laptops and briefcases – a small suitcase on wheels may be the answer.

Dressing tips

✓ To appear friendly and approachable, you need to wear colours of medium depth. Black and other dark shades represent authority, while red makes you appear assertive: *go to pages 28–31*.

✓ To look efficient, your grooming has to be impeccable. If your hair is unwashed, you will give the impression of not caring about yourself. If you haven't applied any make-up, others may think that you're not in control of your time management.

✓ Complete your formal look from head to toe: a tailored suit calls for toned-down accessories, and tights (pantyhose) are essential, whatever the time of year.

✓ Check your look in a mirror before you leave for the office or function: pretend to pick something off the floor and look at what you see – watch out for that cleavage. Sit down, and see how far your skirt rides up.

✓ Showing too much flesh isn't appropriate in a business or formal environment. Exceptionally long nails are also unsuitable.

For advice on what styles will flatter your body shape the most: *go to pages 106–137*; for a selection of key pieces in different styles: *go to pages 126–129*.

Your business look needs to reflect the core values of the industry in which you work

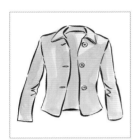

Jacket

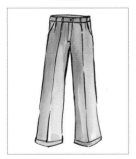

Skirt

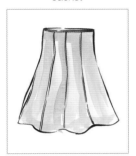

Trousers

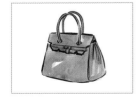

Bag

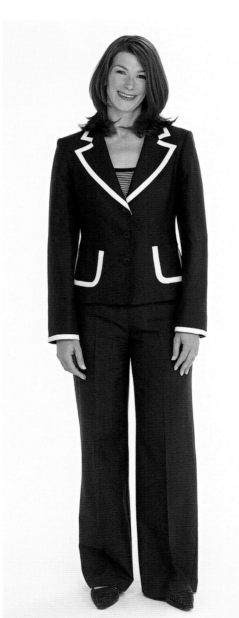

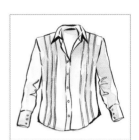

Top

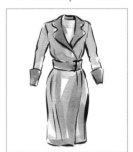

Dress

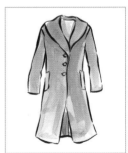

Overcoat

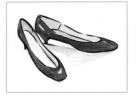

Shoes

Casual capsule

As with your formal wear (pages 184–185), a 'capsule' wardrobe of basic casual pieces that you can mix and match will allow you to put together a number of different outfits without breaking the bank. Remember, though, that a casual look doesn't mean that you don't need to care about your appearance.

Main wardrobe

Jackets or cardigans
Four jackets or cardigans, or perhaps one jacket, two cardigans and one fleece.

Skirts, trousers or jeans
Six of the above – a combination of whichever you prefer and feel most comfortable in.

Tops
Eight tops, from T-shirts to sweaters.

Dresses
These can be substituted for the skirt and top options.

Accessories

Shoes
Four pairs of shoes, boots or trainers.

Bags
Two handbags that complement your lifestyle.

Dressing tips

✓ Maintain the quality and fit of your clothing.

✓ Loose-fitting clothing, provided that it suits your body shape, is perfect for a smart casual look, but make sure that the fabric doesn't cling to your body.

✓ Co-ordinating separates in soft, textured fabrics can replace formal jackets, skirts and trousers.

✓ Give your dresses a different look by teaming them with either a wrap or a cardigan.

✓ Think about separating your formal suits, and wearing the jackets with a casual skirt, pair of trousers or dress.

✗ Dirty, faded, damaged or unkempt clothing isn't acceptable.

For advice on what styles will flatter your body shape the most: *go to pages 106–137*; for a selection of key pieces in different styles: *go to pages 126–129*.

When dressing casually, make sure you don't let your grooming standards slip

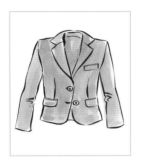

Jacket

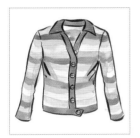

Cardigan

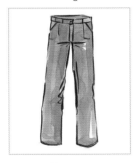

Trousers

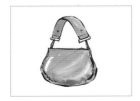

Bag

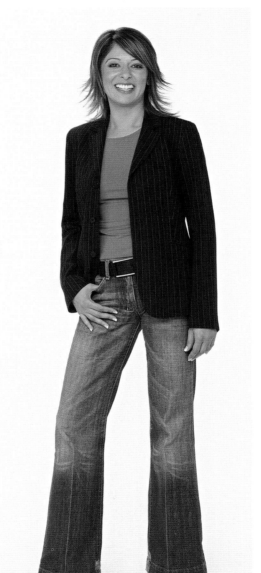

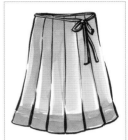

Skirt

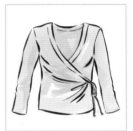

Top

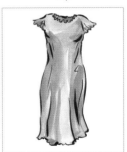

Dress

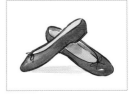

Shoes

Planning for the future

By matching your lifestyle to your wardrobe, you'll end up with more clothes that you actually wear. Create two pie charts, one reflecting your daily activities, the other the contents of your wardrobe. If they don't match up, take action to make your clothes suit your lifestyle with the help of the checklist opposite.

Pie charts

Draw two pie charts. Divide the first chart into sections to reflect the amount of time you spend each day doing the following activities:

Working
At home/looking after children
Social/entertainment
Leisure/hobbies
Errands

Divide the second pie chart into sections to reflect what your wardrobe holds, using the same headings.

If you spend 50% of your time in the office, then 50% of your wardrobe should be represented by your work clothes. Likewise, if you spend only 5% of your time socializing, only 5% of your wardrobe should be for social occasions, and so on.

If the charts don't match, it's time to adjust the balance of your wardrobe so that it reflects your lifestyle.

In the sample charts below, the work clothes outweigh the social and leisure clothes, so any new purchases should be out of work clothes.

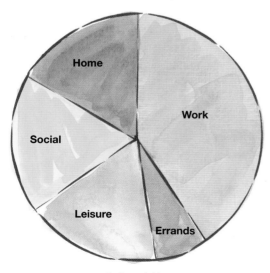

Daily activities

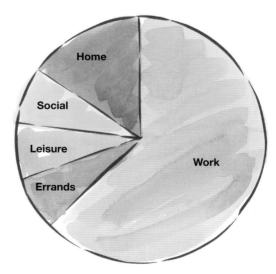

Contents of wardrobe

Checklist

Using the checklist below, note the colour and style of the clothes that you already own. You can then work out the clothes that you need to create your ideal wardrobe. If you wish, make photocopies of the chart to use each time you overhaul your wardrobe. You can also download a more detailed checklist from the **colour me beautiful** website: www.cmb.co.uk

	Colours I have	Styles I have	Colours I need	Styles I need
Jackets				
Skirts				
Trousers				
Tops				
Dresses				
Coats				
Underwear				
Shoes				
Handbags				
Scarves				
Belts				

Index

Acknowledgements

This has been the most fun we have had in our 39 (!!) combined years of working, living and breathing **colour me beautiful**. It would not have been possible without the enthusiasm of the Hamlyn team; everyone there and at Airedale worked so hard. Thank you for putting this baby to bed. We have learned so much from all of you.

We are also grateful to the following: The **colour me beautiful** consultants who checked our improved colour concept: Annie Bucknill, Madge Campbell, Joan Cashman, Melanie Fitzgerald-Power, Julie Houldsworth, Lorna Hudson, Maria Price, and also Angela Wright, FRSA, the colour psychologist.

Our senior European trainers: Helen Allen, Cliff Bashforth and Sue Trevaskis, who made notations on the first draft.

Our consultants and models: Norma Couch, Ros Evans, Micchi Leung, Ruth Murphy, Dipti Patel, Beth Price, Liz Scott, Sue Trevaskis and Mary Watson, who shared the contents of their wardrobes. Mollie Bachman, Camilla Davis, Angela Harris, Ivy Harris, Danni Meharg and Nicole Stephens for their patience in front of the camera.

The kind PRs who lent us clothes for the shoot: Betty Barclay (including Gil Bret and Vera Mount), Jaeger, Hobbs, Kaleidoscope, L.K. Bennett, Sahara, Tu and Wallis. It is wonderful to see all your clothes come alive on real people.

Louise Ravenscroft and Tom Henderson for correcting grammar and Frenchisms.

The team at head office who made sure they avoided us on bad hair days. Audrey Hanna, in particular, kept cool, calm and organized schedules and lists. And, of course, Geoff Thorn, Jill Bay and Mel May, too.

Chris Scarles for his support, encouragement and for letting us take **colour me beautiful** into the new century.

And, finally, our long-suffering husbands, John Henderson and Jim Henshaw, who also live and breathe **colour me beautiful**, and whom we allow the odd sartorial faux pas.

And a big thank you to each other, too.

Veronique Henderson and Pat Henshaw

For more information on services, products and how to become a consultant, contact **colour me beautiful**:

UK and Headquarters for Europe, Africa and the Middle East
66 The Business Centre, 15–17 Ingate Place,
London SW8 3NS
www.colourmebeautiful.co.uk
info@cmb.co.uk
t: +44 (0)20 7627 5211
f: +44 (0)20 7627 5680

Americas and Australasia www.colormebeautiful.com
t: (001) 1-800-606 3435
Austria, France, Germany, Italy, Switzerland & Russia
www.colourmebeautiful.eu
Canada www.colormebeautiful.ca
Finland colormebeautiful@kolumbi.fi
Hong Kong www.colormebeautiful.hk
Ireland www.cmb-ireland.ie
Netherlands & Belgium www.colourmebeautiful.nu
Norway & Denmark www.colormebeautiful.no
Slovenia www.cmb.si
South Africa www.colormebeautiful.co.za
Spain www.cmb-asesoresdeimagen.com
Sweden www.colormebeautiful.se

Picture acknowledgements

Special Photography: © **Octopus Publishing Group Limited**/Mike Prior.
Other photography: **Alamy**/All Star Picture Library 27.
Corbis U.K. Limited/Stephane Cardinale/People Avenue 154; /Najlah Feanny-Hicks/SABA 150; /Frank Trapper 26 centre, 58. **Getty Images** 144; /George DeSota 26 bottom centre, 70; /Jon Kopaloff 26 centre right, 82; /Vanina Lucchesi/Stringer/2005 AFP 26 bottom right, 94; /Gene Shaw 146; /Kevin Winter 26 bottom left, 46, 148. **Rex Features** 27 left; /SRK/Dave Allocca 26 centre left, 32 top, 34; /Startracks (SRK) 152. **TopFoto**/Geoff Caddick 108.

For hamlyn

Executive Editor Sarah Ford
Executive Art Editor Karen Sawyer
Senior Production Controller Manjit Sihra
Picture Researchers Mariana Sonnenburg, Miriam Hyman
Illustrator Kevin Jones Associates
Photographer Mike Prior
Make-up Styling Amanda Cross
Hair Styling Phil Gallagher at Headmasters
www.hmhair.co.uk

Designed and produced by Airedale Publishing Ltd
Project Manager Amanda Jensen
Art Editor Ruth Prentice
Designers Hannah Attwell, Isabel de Cordova
Editors Carole McGlynn, Zia Mattocks, Helen Ridge